Talking together about an autism diagnosis

A guide for parents and carers of children with an autism spectrum disorder

By Rachel Pike, NAS Regional Officer
Illustrated by Jess Abbo

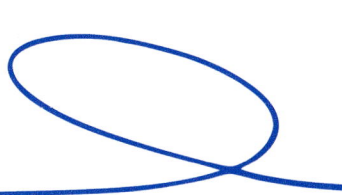

Contents

Introduction	4
To tell or not to tell?	5
When to talk about the diagnosis	7
Autism spectrum disorders (ASDs) and learning difficulties	8
Introducing the subject	9
Who is the best person to talk about the diagnosis?	10
What language should be used?	10
How to talk about the diagnosis	11
What to say	12
Possible reactions	15
What might help if your child rejects their diagnosis	17
Parents' concerns answered by The National Autistic Society *help!* team	19
Who else needs to know?	21
Talking to brothers and sisters	21
Talking to classmates and peers	22
What if your child does not want you to tell other people about the diagnosis?	22
Talking to adults with an ASD about their diagnosis	23
Frequently asked questions	24
Conclusion	27
Appendix one – Worksheet for person with learning difficulties	28
Appendix two – Making a 'Pictures of me' workbook	29
Appendix three – The National Autistic Society worksheet for primary school aged children	35
Appendix four – The National Autistic Society schools lesson plan	39
References	45
Useful resources	46

Talking together about an autism diagnosis

Introduction

This book is aimed primarily at parents and carers of children and young people with an autism spectrum disorder (ASD). Teachers will also find Appendices 3 and 4 particularly useful, as these are aimed at schools.

The book gives some practical tips and strategies for sharing the diagnosis of an ASD with your child or the person you care for. It is also useful for people working with children and young people with an ASD or for people who care for older adolescents or adults on the autism spectrum.

Autism is a spectrum disorder. This means that, while all people with autism share three main areas of difficulty, their condition will affect them in very different ways.

Because it is a spectrum condition, a different approach will be needed for each child, and parents will know best where to pitch their discussion. The resources listed at the end will help in tailoring the discussion for your child.

A note on terminology

Diagnostic terms vary. Your child may have a diagnosis of autism, Asperger syndrome, an ASD, pervasive development disorder (PDD) or something else. These tips and strategies will apply to anyone who has one of these diagnoses. Some of the books and other resources quoted may use a specific term. If you are going to use this resource with the person you are supporting it may help to go through and insert the diagnostic term that is appropriate to them. Some people with an ASD may interpret things very literally – if something refers to autism and they have a diagnosis of Asperger syndrome, they may find it difficult to believe it can apply to them as well. For consistency, however, the abbreviation ASD is used throughout the book.

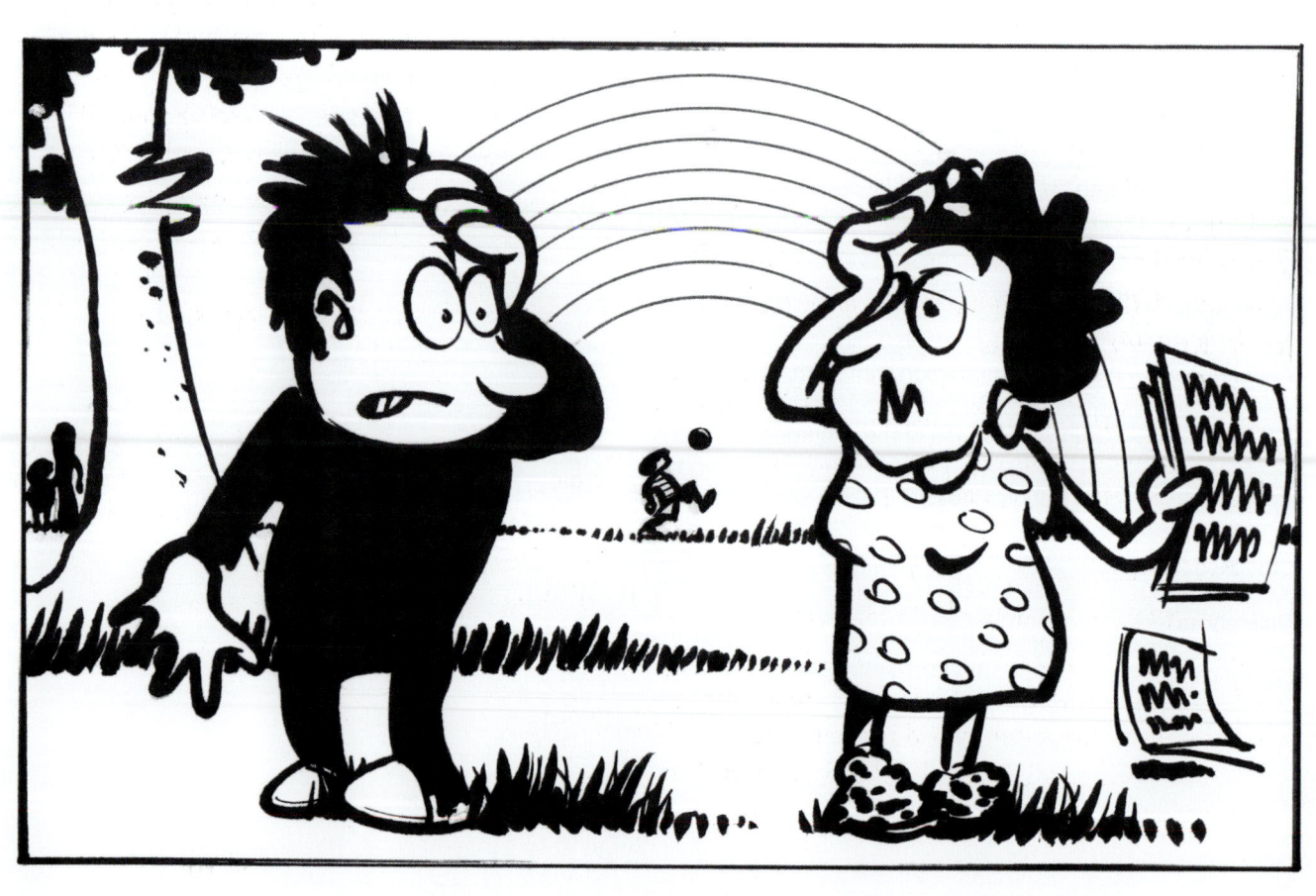

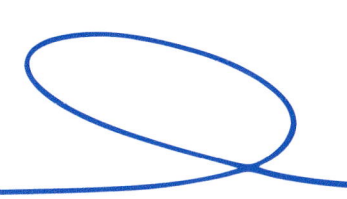

To tell or not to tell?

A person who has an ASD has a right to know their diagnosis. Wanting to protect them from the diagnosis can feel like the kindest thing to do, but in reality it often gets harder the longer it is delayed. There are definite advantages to talking about the diagnosis with your child but these will vary between individuals. Many people who have an ASD have commented that they would have liked to have been told about their diagnosis earlier because knowing came as a relief and a source of comfort.

Here are some of the possible advantages of talking about the diagnosis with your child.

> It can help them to make sense of their difficulties and know that it is not their fault, that there is a reason and a name for their difficulties. This can come as a relief to some people who might have felt that they were the only person to struggle in certain situations.
> They may find out anyway by overhearing you or someone else using the term and draw their own (perhaps misguided) conclusions.
> They may be aware that they are going to visit the doctor for assessments and may draw the wrong conclusions from these visits, such as thinking that they are ill.
> It can help ensure suitable provision is found as they get older – for example, declaring an ASD when applying for a college place means that extra support could be available to enable them to achieve their academic potential.
> By being open about the diagnosis you can agree who else needs to know and ensure that teachers, peers, colleagues, support staff, etc have the right information.
> There is a growing network of contacts and support for people with an ASD – much of it is online and set up by people with a similar diagnosis. By knowing their diagnosis, your child can talk to other people who think and act in the same way and may even share the same interests.
> The right help and support could enable your child to advocate for him or herself.
> There are also ethical issues: an individual has a right to know – wouldn't you want to know the results of a test or an assessment that you have been through?

Parents and carers often worry about some of the potential negative consequences of talking to their child about their diagnosis, for example, people not understanding, the child feeling a failure because they have an ASD or using it as an excuse for certain behaviours. Some of these concerns are considered later in the book but it is worth pointing out that some of these potential negative experiences could still happen even if your child is not told about their diagnosis.

If you are worried about whether or not to tell your child about their diagnosis, it may be helpful to talk to other people who know your child, for example, a supportive professional, family member or friend of the family, and ask their opinion. It is also worth thinking about your own feelings and concerns about the diagnosis and what it might mean for your child and asking yourself whether these may be holding you back. Writing down some of the possible advantages and disadvantages of talking about it may help you.

For some people, getting the diagnosis has been helpful:

'I never understood why I didn't like change – it would have helped me to know that it was to do with my autism and that other people (with autism) hate it too.'
(Doherty, K. et al 2003, p.32)

Talking together about an autism diagnosis

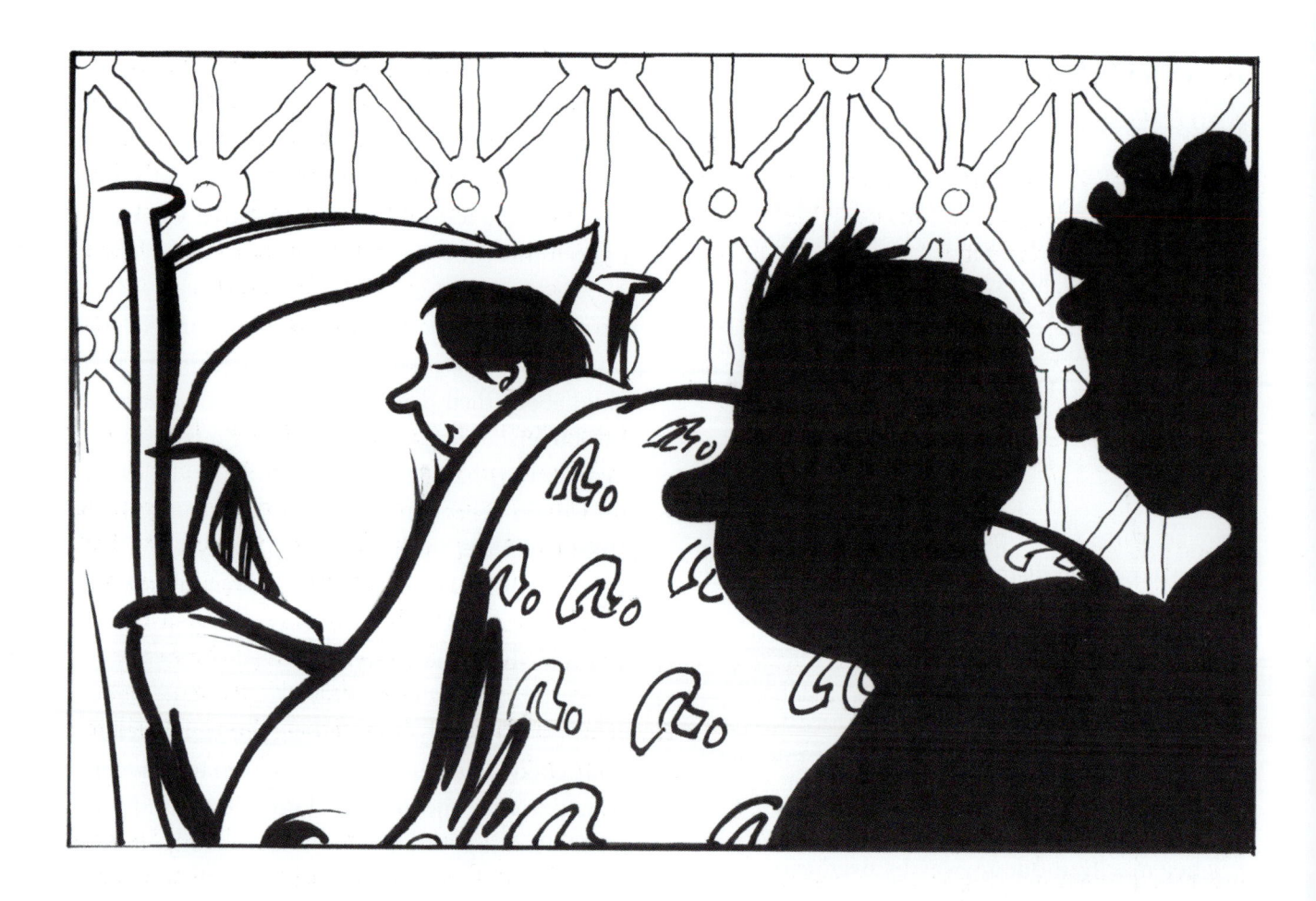

'I had finally found the reason why other people classed me as weird. It was not just because I was clumsy or stupid. My heart lightened instantly and the constant nagging that accompanied me all my life (not my mum) stopped immediately. I finally knew why I felt different, why I felt as though I was a freak, why I didn't seem to fit in. Even better it was not my fault! So my final word on this subject is get them told!'
(Jackson L. 2002, pp. 34-37)

'Getting the label was one of the best things that has ever happened to me. By my teens I was seriously depressed after years of being different and not knowing why. When I didn't have an official diagnostic label, my teachers unofficially labelled me as emotionally disturbed, rude and so on, and my classmates labelled me as weirdo, freak and nerd. Frankly I prefer the official label.' (Sainsbury C. 2000, p.31)

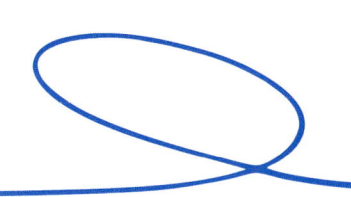

When to talk about the diagnosis

The needs of your child will vary according to their age, ability and specific circumstances. Their diagnosis may mean that their level of understanding or ability to process language is different to other children their age, so the right time or age to discuss the diagnosis will depend on their individual abilities, needs and emotional strength. The language you use to discuss it will also need to be pitched according to your child's age and understanding.

It won't be a one-off conversation – it is something that you will need to come back to, and different words and resources will need to be used at different times. Being open and honest from the outset can help in the longer term.

Some children and young people will need and want to be involved with the diagnostic process right from the start. Others will not feel able to be involved at the beginning and may find it a lot harder to come to terms with. Continuing to be open and honest with the child and young person as much as possible along the way can help.

Some parents and carers have found that the right time for this conversation has been when their child has started to ask questions about why they are different from the other children in their class – why they get extra help or find it difficult to make friends. But be aware that the nature of an ASD means that some individuals may have worries but find it difficult to express them.

Some children and young people will already have additional diagnoses, for example, dyspraxia and dyslexia, and so explanations about a diagnosis of an ASD can follow on from those already given about these previous diagnoses.

Tony Attwood says, "There is no simple answer. Very young children will not have the maturity to understand the concepts. Older children may be extremely sensitive to any suggestion that they are different… The answer may be to tell the child when they are emotionally able to cope with the information and want to know why they have difficulties in situations that other children find so easy. Sometimes this should be undertaken by parents, sometimes by a professional." (Attwood T. 1998, p.178)

Generally it will not be the right time for you to talk about an ASD until you feel that you can explain the condition positively and when you are confident that you can answer any questions that come up or at least know where to go to find out the answer. If the subject remains a sensitive issue for you as a parent or carer, it might be worth thinking about whether there is a trusted family member, friend or professional who could talk to your child.

Some studies have suggested that adolescents with an ASD can find it particularly hard to accept a new diagnosis or may even reject a previously accepted diagnosis. However, individuals often go on to accept the diagnosis after the particular difficulties associated with adolescence have passed. So, if possible, try to have the discussion well before your child reaches adolescence.

For some children and young people, a knowledge of the diagnosis may give rise to more problems that outweigh the potential benefits of knowing. For example, it may more harmful for them to know if they are going through a period of particular stress, anxiety or change. In these situations, it is important to talk through some of these issues with the professionals who are working with your child, so that you have all agreed whether or not it is the right time to talk about the diagnosis. You know your child the best, so you will be able to judge what is in his or her best interest.

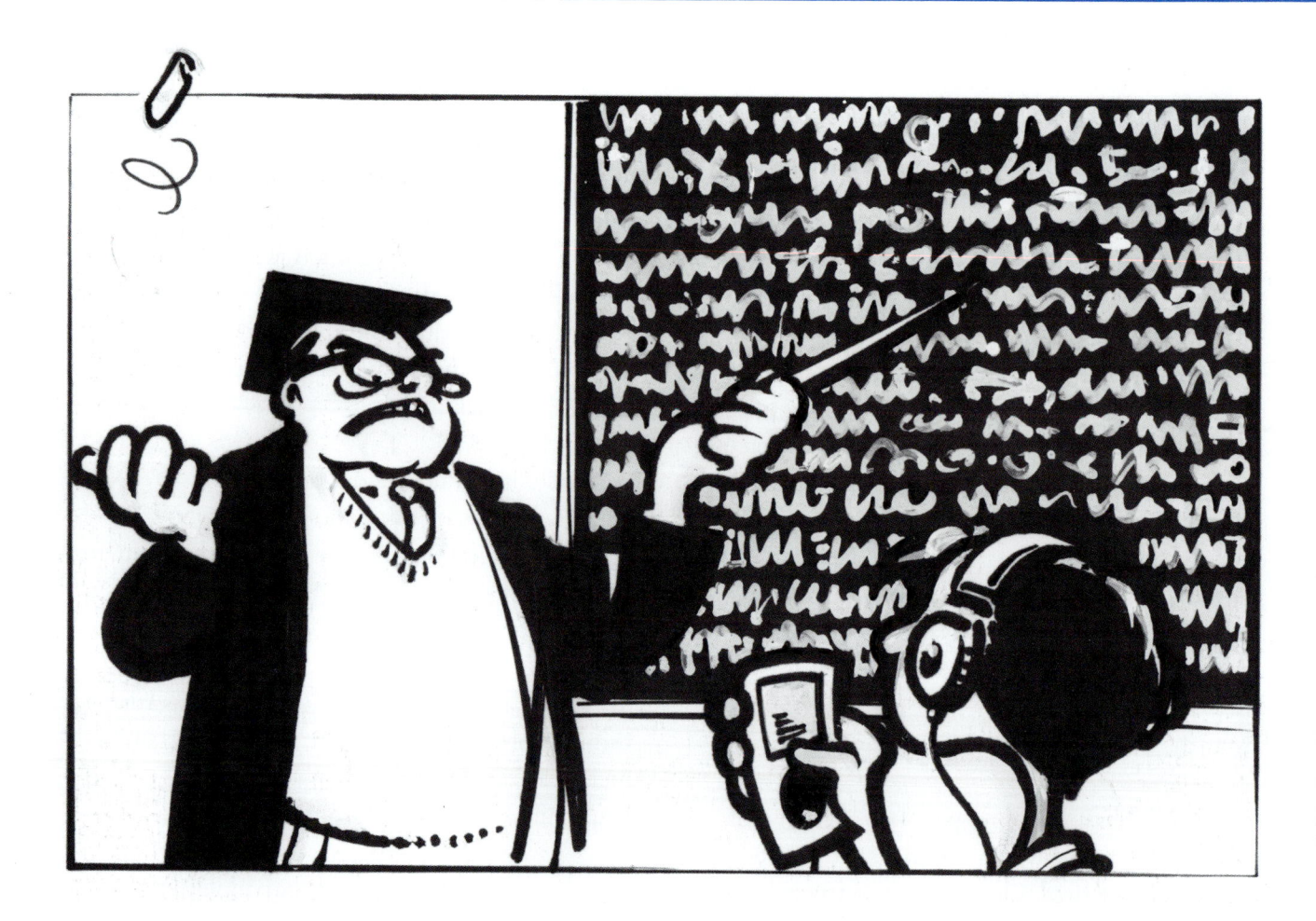

ASDs and learning difficulties

For children with an ASD and learning difficulties, it will be useful to identify strategies for talking about ASDs using words and pictures that will be more meaningful for them. See appendix 1 for an easy to follow sheet to explain the diagnosis. Glenys Jones talks about parents or carers of people with an ASD and learning difficulties drawing up 'passports' or manuals which list the things that the individual enjoys, as well as the areas they need particular support with. These would be written from the perspective of the child or young person and would help the reader to have insight into how an ASD affects that individual. (Jones G. 2001, p65-71)

For children with learning difficulties, it can be particularly important to use language, words and communication styles which suit them. Adapting some of the books and resources aimed at a younger age group to make them more appropriate could be useful.

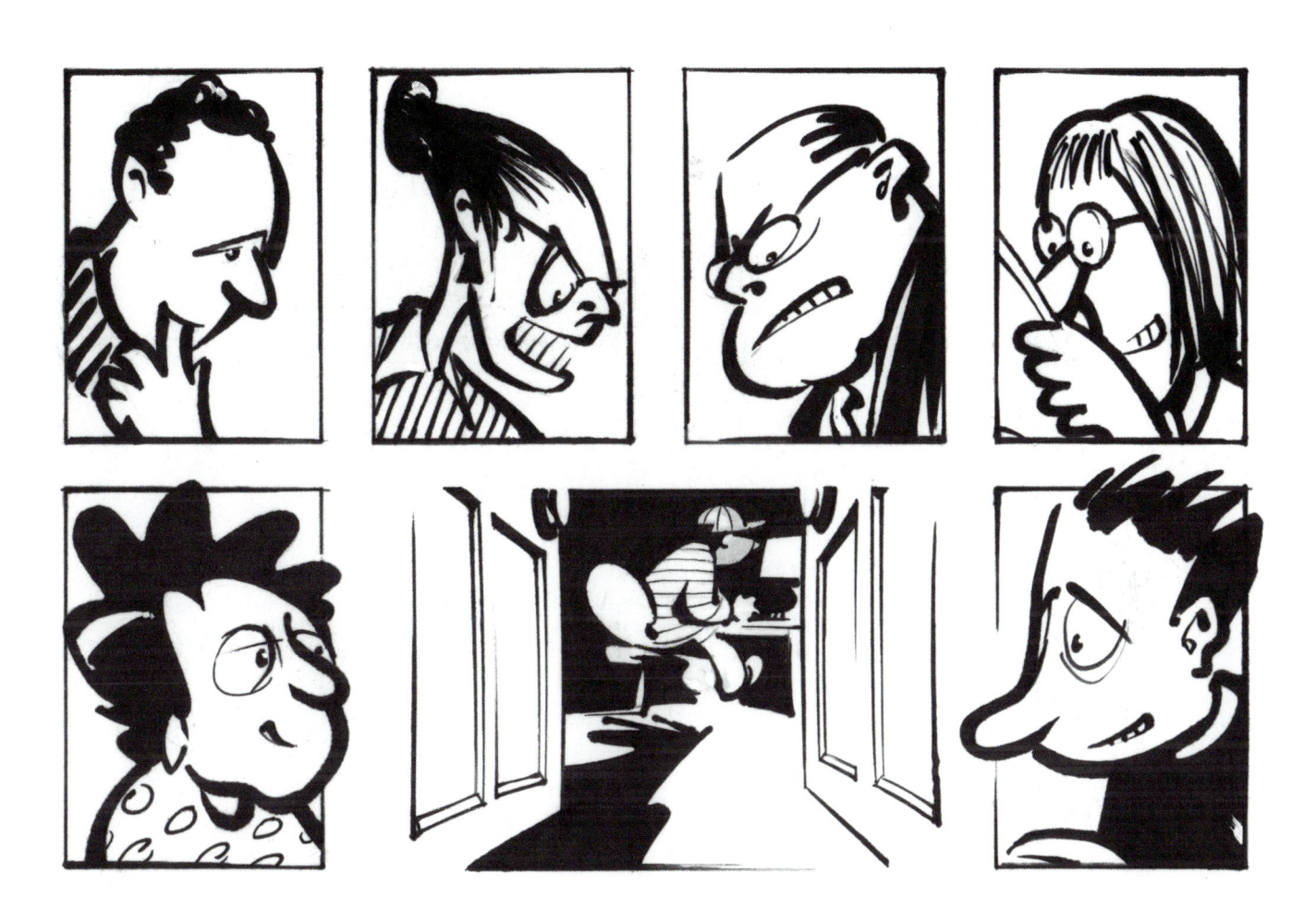

Introducing the subject

This will vary for each individual. It might feel like the right time is after an appointment or meeting. Some parents have seized the moment after attending a talk about ASDs, when they feel more confident and knowledgeable about the diagnosis. The discussion may arise naturally after an incident at school which relates to their ASD.

Christopher Gillberg talks about a young boy who came into his office and by chance picked up a leaflet about an ASD and realised that it was something that related to him. (Gillberg C. 1991, p138) Several parents have reported how they left information out for their child, who picked it up themselves. For these young people it may have been the right approach as the parents said that the child would struggle to accept something directly from them.

If a natural opportunity does not arise and you plan to sit down with your child, here are some tips about creating the right environment to do so.

> It might be useful to visit a local support group and meet other parents of children with an ASD to hear about how they introduced the subject to their child. It might also be useful to take your child along to a family session so that he or she will know there are other people with a similar profile of difficulties and abilities.
> Doing some background work beforehand might help – talking about the differences in the family and celebrating each person's differences can prepare the ground for talking about an ASD.
> Ensure the young person is relaxed and that there are no other distractions – trying to talk about the diagnosis whilst they are on the PlayStation will not be successful!

Talking together about an autism diagnosis

> If there is a time of day that is better for your child – or an environment in which they are particularly relaxed – then use that.
> Be sure that you will be around if there are any follow up questions.
> Ensure you have resources, etc to hand.

Who is the best person to talk about the diagnosis?

In general it is parents and carers, or the person who conducted the diagnosis, who talk to the child about the diagnosis. But other people can be just as helpful and in some cases more appropriate.

Some children or young people would prefer to hear it straight from the GP/diagnostician. In this way, if they have any questions, these can be answered knowledgeably. This might also be a preferred option if as a parent you are still struggling to understand the diagnosis and what it means for your child. Some parents also report that their child often finds it hard to accept what they say but may accept it from someone else.

Again there might be a trusted professional or friend of the family who you feel would be more appropriate. Some professionals are skilled in this type of work and can talk about the diagnosis sensitively and positively. This can also help the young person not to blame you as a parent for the diagnosis – you can be there to give support and answer any questions that might come up afterwards. However it is important that you as a parent have confidence that the professional is able to talk to your child in the right way.

If there is a professional who you feel would be the right person to talk to your child – such as a specialist ASD family support worker, a youth worker, a teacher or a community nurse – ensure that they have a good grasp of the condition and how it might affect your child. Also ensure that they can answer any other questions that may arise and that the language they use is positive and up to date.

What language should be used?

Use language that your child understands. It is important when talking about the diagnosis that the language is right for your child. Be sure that any technical terms you use are up to date as this is the language that your child will hear outside of the home. It is important to use common language and not any family words for the condition, as this may confuse him or her later. Remember that your child's literal understanding may mean that if someone uses a different label for their condition they will not necessarily understand that they are talking about the same condition. For some children the diagnostic terms will be fairly meaningless; it will be the words to explain it which will be more valuable.

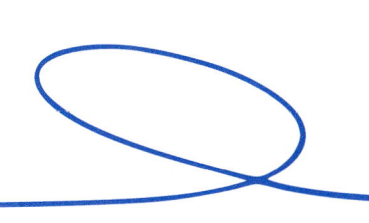

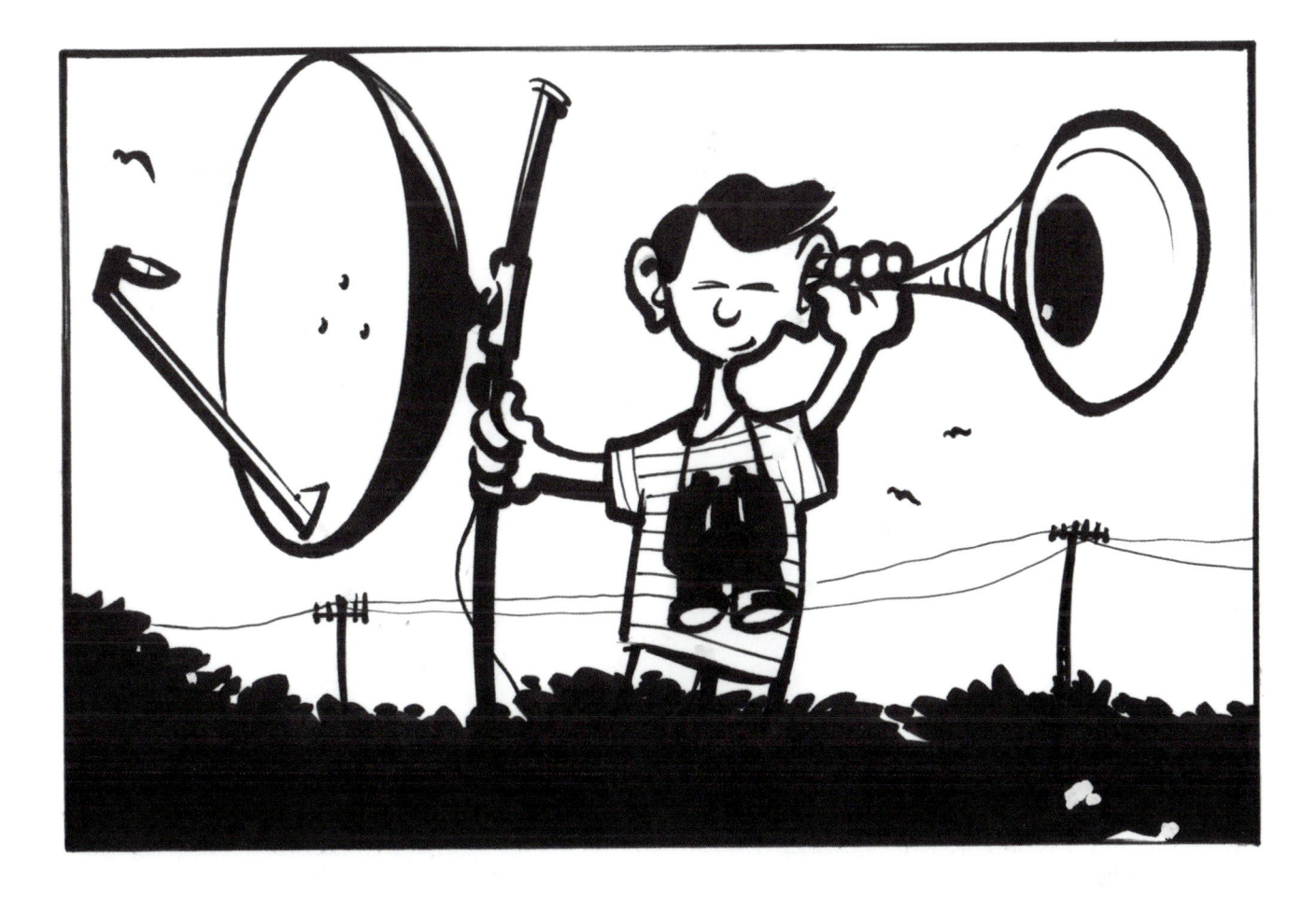

How to talk about the diagnosis

Identify the most suitable communication method

People with ASDs often respond better to different methods of communication. What might work for you as a person without an ASD may be very different to what is right for your child. It might be that talking about it is most helpful, but writing it down, writing an email, drawing pictures, using comic strips etc could also be just as – or even more – effective. There are lots of books and resources available which can help with this.

Some families have found using Carol Gray's Social Stories™ (Gray C. 2002) approach useful. There is more information about Social Stories on her website – see references at end. There are also courses run on Social Stories around the country that might be useful for you to attend (go to www.autismdirectory.org.uk for details).

'Pictures of Me' is a Social Story that introduces an individual to their diagnosis of an ASD. It is put together with the individual, parents and/or professionals and talks about the child's personality, particular strengths and talents as well as some of the things they might find difficult. An example is reproduced at the end of this book (see Appendix 2).

The needs and abilities of children, young people and adults with an ASD vary hugely. Methods and approaches which work for one individual do not necessarily work for another. Try to identify a communication method that works well for your child or the person you are working with. Many people with an ASD need visual information as well as verbal information. Many people have difficulties processing what is being said, so having information, books etc to back up what you are saying can be useful.

Talking together about an autism diagnosis

Link it to special interests

If your child has a special interest, think about how this could be used, for example, if they like Harry Potter, talking about Harry Potter's strengths and weaknesses before talking about your child's. One young person with an ASD was able to make his own analogy when he said, "So it's kind of like the Muggles in Harry Potter."

Another parent linked the discussion to her son's fascination with electricity and said having an ASD could be compared to being wired up differently.

Think about how much information to give

It is important not to give too much information the first time you talk about ASDs. You will know your child and how much information they can deal with. As mentioned above, it is worth having some additional resources prepared as back-ups in case they have further questions. For example, DVDs about ASDs, books, useful websites etc. Be sure to let them know they can ask further questions at any time.

General pointers

> - The longer you put it off, the harder it can get.
> - But... ensure you feel positive and confident about the diagnosis before sharing it with your child.
> - Individual needs about when, where, how much information etc will vary.
> - Talking about an ASD to your child is an ongoing process. They may want to talk more about it immediately or at some point in the future, or may need to keep coming back to it.
> - Reassure them that you will answer any questions that they want to ask, and that you can talk about it more in the future if they would like to.
> - It might be useful to think about contacting other people with an ASD, so that your child can meet other people with a similar diagnosis. Our Autism Helpline (0845 070 4004, Mon-Fri, 10am-4pm) can put you in touch with local groups and organisations.
> - Be prepared for your child to 'close down' the discussion. This may be due to lack of interest or understanding or it may be a case of information overload. Be prepared to return to the discussion in the future or to take a different approach.

What to say

It is important to keep the tone of the conversation positive and to emphasise that everyone has differences: stress that there are things that we are good at as well as things we find hard. (It could be helpful to have prepared some examples to illustrate this.)

Here are some tips that have helped other people – there is not just one way to talk about ASDs.

One parent said she heard a talk about ASDs and decided to tell her nine-year-old son straightaway afterwards. On the way home in the car she said to her son, "You know how you talk about feeling that there are things you do differently to other children? Well, there is a name for that, it is called autism. It's OK to do things differently because I do things differently too and I am OK." She reported that her son was quite happy with this explanation and later began to talk about having an ASD.

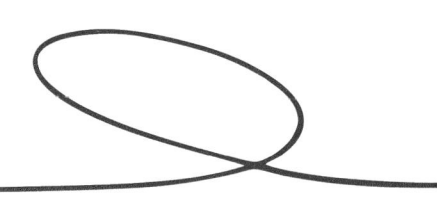

Some parents like to write out an explanation. Here is one way that a parent explained Asperger syndrome to her six-year-old son:

I am special
I am a very special person. I am very clever and good at doing lots of things:

Some things I do well	Some things I find difficult	Mummy, daddy and my teachers will always try to help me with the things that I find difficult. Quite a lot of people (some famous) have a brain as special as mine. The special name for how I am is Asperger syndrome. People cannot see Asperger syndrome because it is inside my brain. I am loved by lots of people and I am able to make many people happy with my kindness.
Reading	Changes	
Writing	Looking at people's faces	
Drawing	Knowing how I feel	
Using computers		
Remembering things		

Think about making a scrapbook or collage with your child beforehand which clearly shows all the things they are good at and enjoy, as well as the things they find difficult.

Here are some of the kind of things that could be included.

My name is Joe. I am eight years old. I live with my mum, my dad and my sister.

I really love swimming and dinosaurs.

I am good at computers. I am very honest. Teachers at school say that I am very reliable. Mum says that I am good at keeping my bedroom tidy.

I can get upset sometimes when things don't go to plan.

I find it hard to understand why my sister makes so much noise sometimes.

At school my handwriting needs more practice than some of the other children.

The reason I find some things hard, but am good at other things is because I have Asperger syndrome.

Asperger syndrome was first written about by a man called Hans Asperger. He described some children that were like me as well. Everybody is different and everybody is good at some things and not so good at other things. My brain works differently to lots of other people. But there is nothing wrong with it. Some other people's brains also work like mine. In history some of the people who are very famous had brains who work in similar ways to mine. Some people think these people might have had Asperger syndrome.

Talking together about an autism diagnosis

General tips for what to say

> Keep explanations about an ASD simple. Think about what your child needs to know at this point. You could give further information at a later stage.
> Think in advance about what you want to say. It may help to write it down beforehand so that you have your own prompts or script.
> Keep language positive.
> Talk about what your child **can** do as well as what they need extra help with. For example, say, "you have a different way of talking to people," rather than, "you are not very good at talking to people". Talk about the positives – that we need people with an ASD because they can help teach us to see the world differently and can come up with new ideas. Talk about some of the high-profile people who are thought to have had an ASD. The book *Different like me – my book of autism heroes* may be useful here – see Useful resources, p46
> Talk about everyone being different – with things they are good at, as well as things they need more help with.
> Where appropriate, try to use the term 'difference' rather than 'difficulties'.
> Remember that your child may not know how to voice their concerns, so be sure to stress that it is not their fault, it's not catching and it doesn't get worse. Jackie Jackson writes about a man with Asperger syndrome who knew early on that he had autism but assumed it was his fault so ignored it until he was 16, when he found out it wasn't his fault after all. (Jackson J. 2002, p.120)
> As mentioned above, many people with an ASD respond better to visual information than oral. You might have spent a fair amount of time preparing a speech which you feel happy with but, when you deliver it, your child may find it hard to process what has been said. They may need it backed up with pictures, illustrations etc.
> Help your child to think about the ways in

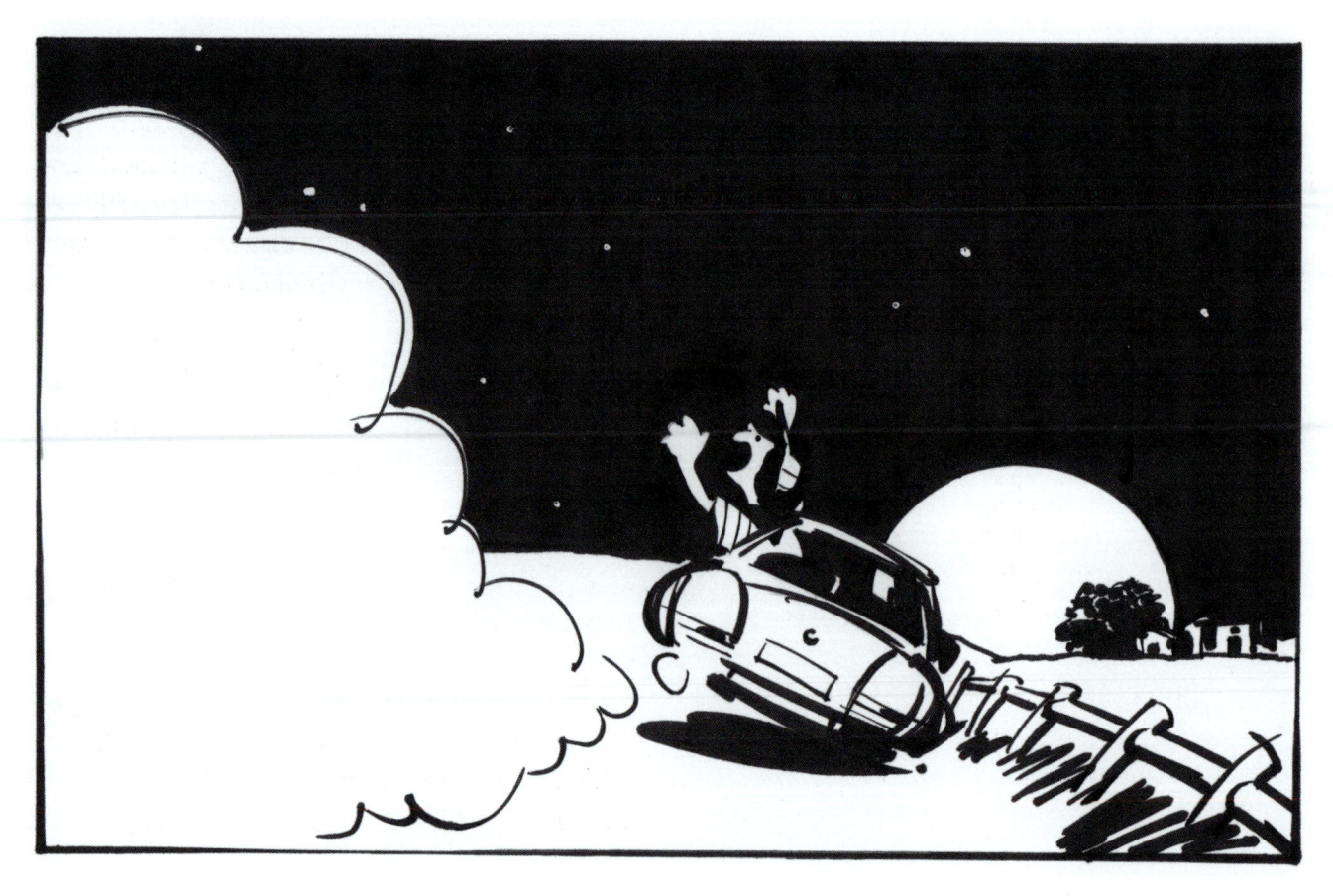

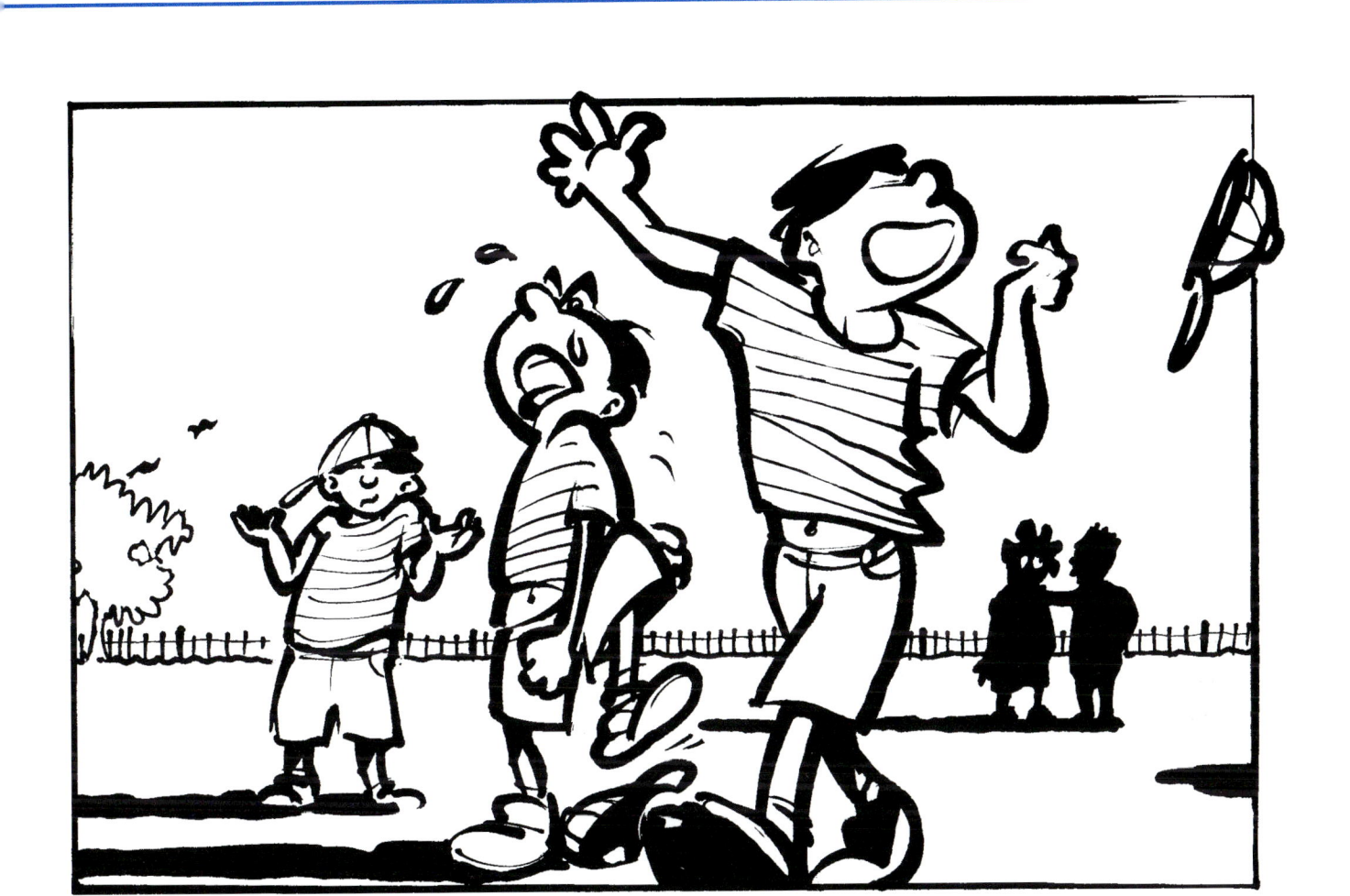

which they are the same as other people as well as the ways that they are different.

> Be aware of the possible literal nature of your child. For example, if you use a book, make sure that it is appropriate for their diagnosis. For example, a child with a diagnosis of Asperger syndrome may feel that the book *I have autism… what's that?* (see Useful resources, p46) does not relate to them.
> Be sure to point out that you do not have to have every characteristic of an ASD for the diagnosis still to apply.
> More able children may want to know lots of details, in particular, how their diagnosis might affect them now and in the future and how it is caused.
> Look at leaflets/information sheets etc aimed at young people or siblings and adapt the language to suit your child.

Possible reactions

Reactions to the diagnosis will vary with each individual. Several parents have reported being very worried about the diagnosis and then pleasantly surprised by their child's immediate acceptance or their seeming lack of interest or concern.

It can be harder for teenagers to accept the diagnosis, as they are struggling with so much else and wanting to fit in. For some the diagnosis can be a particular blow. But for others who have struggled throughout their school life, it can come as relief to realise that there is a name for the things they have been struggling with and, even better, that there are other people out there who are struggling with similar issues.

Your child may react very differently to how you think you would have reacted or to how you yourself responded to finding out their diagnosis.

Talking together about an autism diagnosis

Remember that your child experiences the world and processes information differently to you. They may get upset by some aspect of the diagnosis that would not necessarily concern you or may have completely unexpected questions or concerns. You may be worrying about the future and what this might hold for your child, but they may be more concerned about whether this means they can still play on their PlaysStation that evening!

Some children and adults with an ASD will deny that they have any difficulties and will not accept the diagnosis of an ASD. Arguing about it is usually unhelpful. They will need to come round to the fact in their own time. For some older adolescents or adults who have had incorrect diagnoses in the past, it can be particularly difficult for them to trust yet another diagnosis. A knowledgeable 'expert' in ASDs may be a good person for the individual to see to talk through the various diagnoses and to explain why this one is now thought to be correct.

Do not to get too fixed on the ASD term, if that is what is causing distress to your child. It may be more helpful to work with them to identify the areas they need help and support with, as well as making sure they are reminded of the things they do well. For example, they may not want to accept their diagnosis of an ASD but may feel able to say to people, "I find it hard to understand people if they use too many words when they talk. Could you try to use fewer words?"

Some children will not want to use the term autism or Asperger syndrome but may say of themselves that they have 'communication difficulties' or 'language difficulties'. However, these phrases may not fully describe an individual's difficulties and in some circumstances may be too vague to be helpful.

One family say that their son will not accept the 'A' word, but will accept people being told about his diagnosis and the help and support that can be put in place, as long as no one mentions the word in his presence.

"…where the person's initial response is anger, this does not necessarily indicate that it was wrong to introduce him or her to the diagnosis. The first discussion is but the start of an ongoing process of gradually explaining the underlying reasons for their behaviour, difficulties and strengths. The explanations and discussions can be frequently returned to when opportunities present themselves… The person's initial response might not be their eventual reaction and their comments and feelings on being given the diagnosis can serve as future areas to work on and discuss."
(Jones G. 2001, p.68)

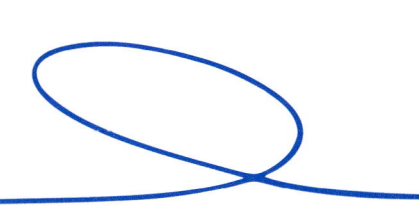

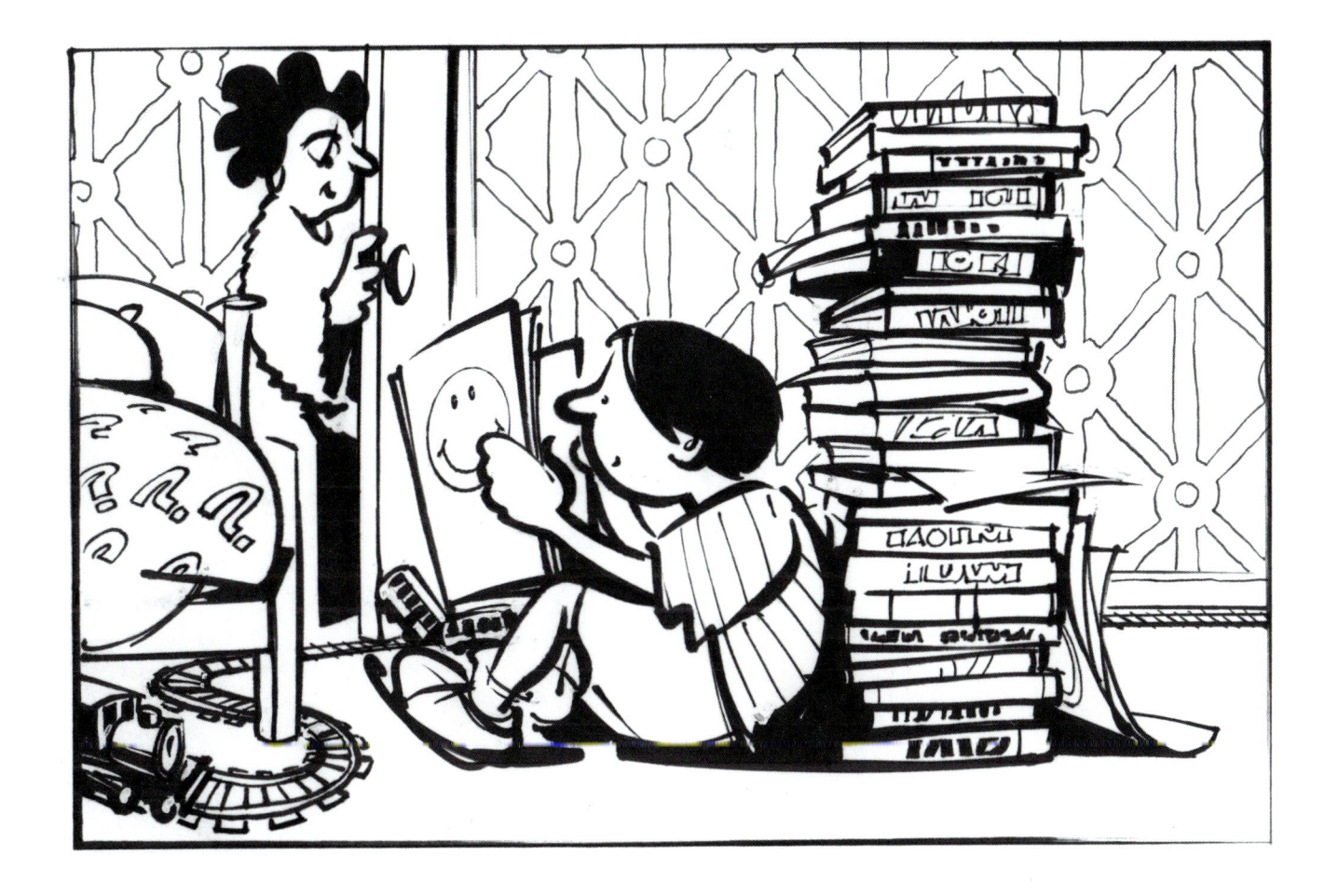

What might help if your child rejects their diagnosis?

You cannot force someone to accept the diagnosis. It may be that they come to accept it over time or, if your child continues to reject the diagnosis completely, that the diagnosis could be used to help inform your interaction with them without talking openly about it.

Everyone will make their own adjustment to knowing that they have an ASD. If the diagnosis is handled positively by the people around your child, this may help them to come to terms with the diagnosis in the longer term.

Allow some time after initially talking about the diagnosis and, if they still reject it, some of the following tips might help:

> Use some of the workbooks and other resources which are now available to go through the diagnosis and what it might mean for them as an individual eg. *I am special* or *what is Asperger syndrome and how will it affect me?* (see Useful resources p46).
> Draw from some of the positive examples of individuals and their achievements so that they know that there can be positives attached to having an ASD. *Different like me* is very helpful (see Useful resources p46).
> Leave personal accounts or information out for your child to pick up and read from as and when they feel inclined, so that they can come to it on their own terms.
> Try to arrange an opportunity for your child to meet with other older, positive people with an ASD who could talk to them about their experiences.

Talking together about an autism diagnosis

> Don't get too fixed on the label – it may be that they will accept the areas they have difficulties with (and accept help and support with these areas) but not the actual term.
> There are some storybooks (eg *Blue bottle mystery* – see Useful resources p46) with positive heroes with an ASD available. If your child enjoys reading stories, these could help provide a positive portrayal of an ASD.
> *Asperger United*, a quarterly magazine produced by people with Asperger syndrome for people with Asperger syndrome provides a good way to learn about others' experiences of living with the condition. (See Useful resources p46).

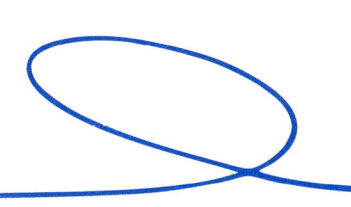

Concerns answered by The National Autistic Society *help!* team

The National Autistic Society *help!* team work with families of older children who have an ASD diagnosis. Here are some typical situations and tips from the team.

"We don't want to tell him while things are going well for him. It might set him back or make him depressed."

It is for each parent to decide their own particular 'right' time but experience suggests that most parents feel it was a good idea to talk about the diagnosis, regardless of whether their child was going through a good or bad patch.

It is possible that your child may react with anger or become stressed as they come to terms with their diagnosis but it may still be important that they know about it.

"I am worried that my son will use the term autism as an excuse for poor behaviour."

One girl said, "Because of my autism I cannot help swearing the words just come out before I can stop to think."

This is not an excuse but an explanation that gives you something to work with. Because this girl knows about her difficulties and is willing to talk about them, it allows her parents to think up strategies to manage. This could simply mean trying to reduce stressful situations for her, learning to count to ten, working out a reward scheme for not swearing or practising less offensive words to use when stressed.

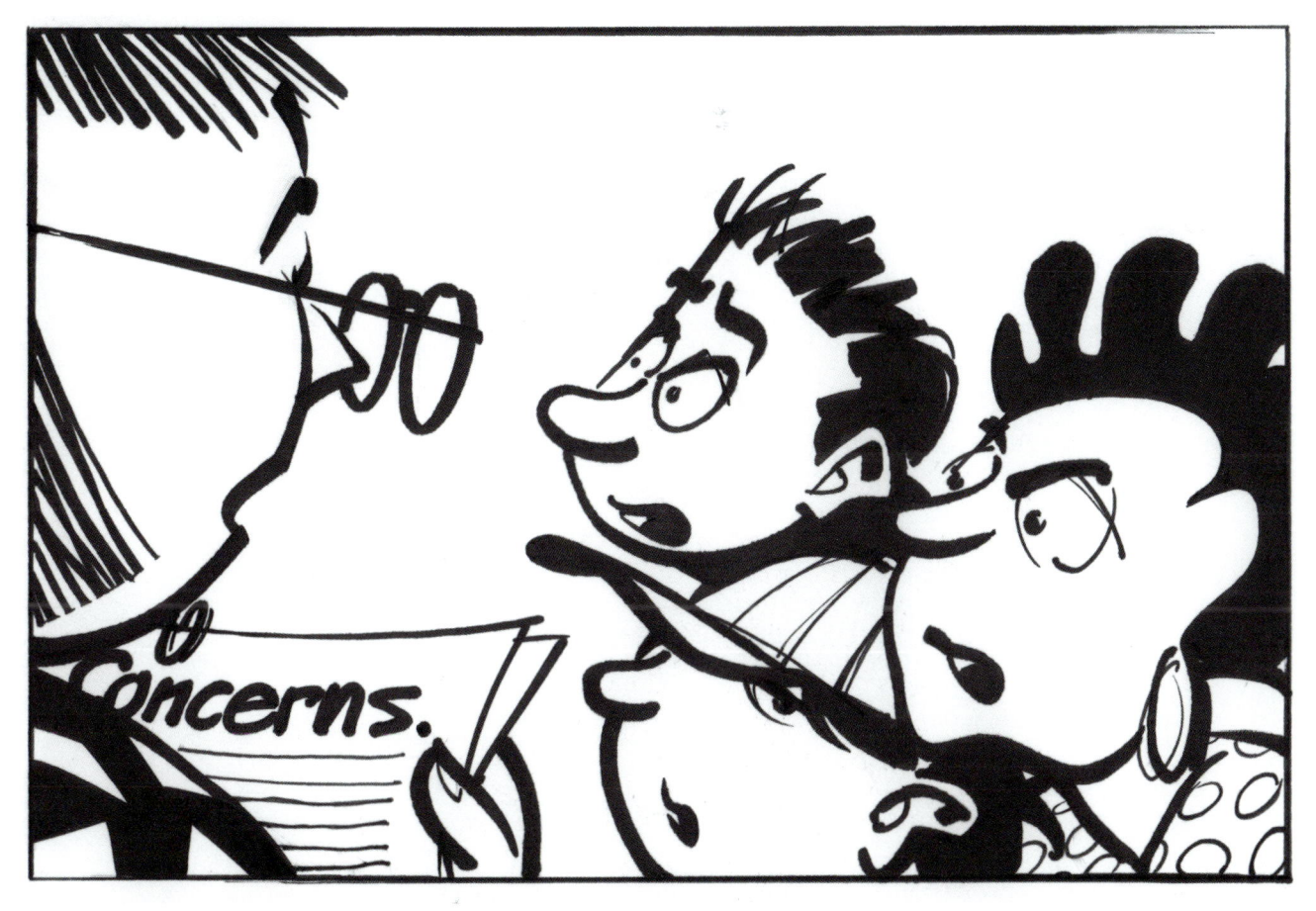

Talking together about an autism diagnosis

If you think your child is just making an excuse, then agree that the task in hand is difficult but that you expect them to get on with the request. Be positive – the fact that they have an ASD does often make life harder, but it also means that they deserve more regular praise for overcoming their difficulties.

Children will often find excuses for not doing something they don't want to do! If they don't blame their difficulties on their diagnosis they'll probably find something else to blame. Generally it doesn't seem to happen as often as parents fear it might. One parent who came to the NAS *help!* programme told the group about their 11-yearold son who told them, "The only known cure for an ASD is a MacDonald's and the occasional Chinese."

"We don't want him to be labelled as disabled because then people will start treating him differently"

This is an understandable worry but also why it is important to explain ASDs to your child, alongside a discussion about who to tell about the diagnosis.

This may include talking about how much the general public understands ASDs, so your child, isn't given a false impression.

Some parents say that they tell other people on a need-to-know basis. Others talk about measuring the costs and benefits of telling each person. Your child may not wish to tell a friend who lives locally, but may wish to tell their classmates. Or they may wish to tell their employer but not their keep fit class.

It may be worth considering that people do treat those with an ASD differently, whether they have a diagnosis or not. People will pick up on the social difficulties and come to their own – often unkind – conclusions about why your child is behaving differently to everyone else.

It is also true to say that being treated 'differently' is often a good thing. We know that people with an ASD do benefit from being treated differently, if that means the other person takes an imaginative step into their world and communicates in a way that is understandable to them.

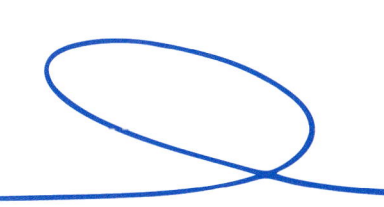

Who else needs to know?

After you have talked about ASDs with your child, it is often helpful to talk about who else needs to know. People to think about would be brothers and sisters, wider family, school staff and neighbours, employers and college lecturers. You can talk together about who should be told and what they should be told.

There is a range of information available to help other people understand, from very brief leaflets to books: the level of information needed will vary with different people and in different settings. See Useful resources p46.

Talking to brothers and sisters

Brothers and sisters may have picked up that there is something going on and, as has been mentioned earlier, may draw the wrong conclusions. They may also be struggling with aspects of their sibling's behaviour, so it can help to talk through the diagnosis with them as well. There are several books, pamphlets, websites and resources available which are specifically aimed at siblings (see Useful resources p46).

It is important that brothers and sisters are given information about an ASD – what it means for their brother or sister, but, just as importantly, what it means for them.

Brothers and sisters will need to know it is not catching and that it is not their fault. They will also need reassurance that they can be honest about their feelings. For example, it is okay to get angry if your brother or sister throws their things across the floor if they are cross. They will need to know that they can come to you to talk about it whenever they want to, that they can ask whatever questions they want, and that, if you don't know the answer at the time you will try to find it out.

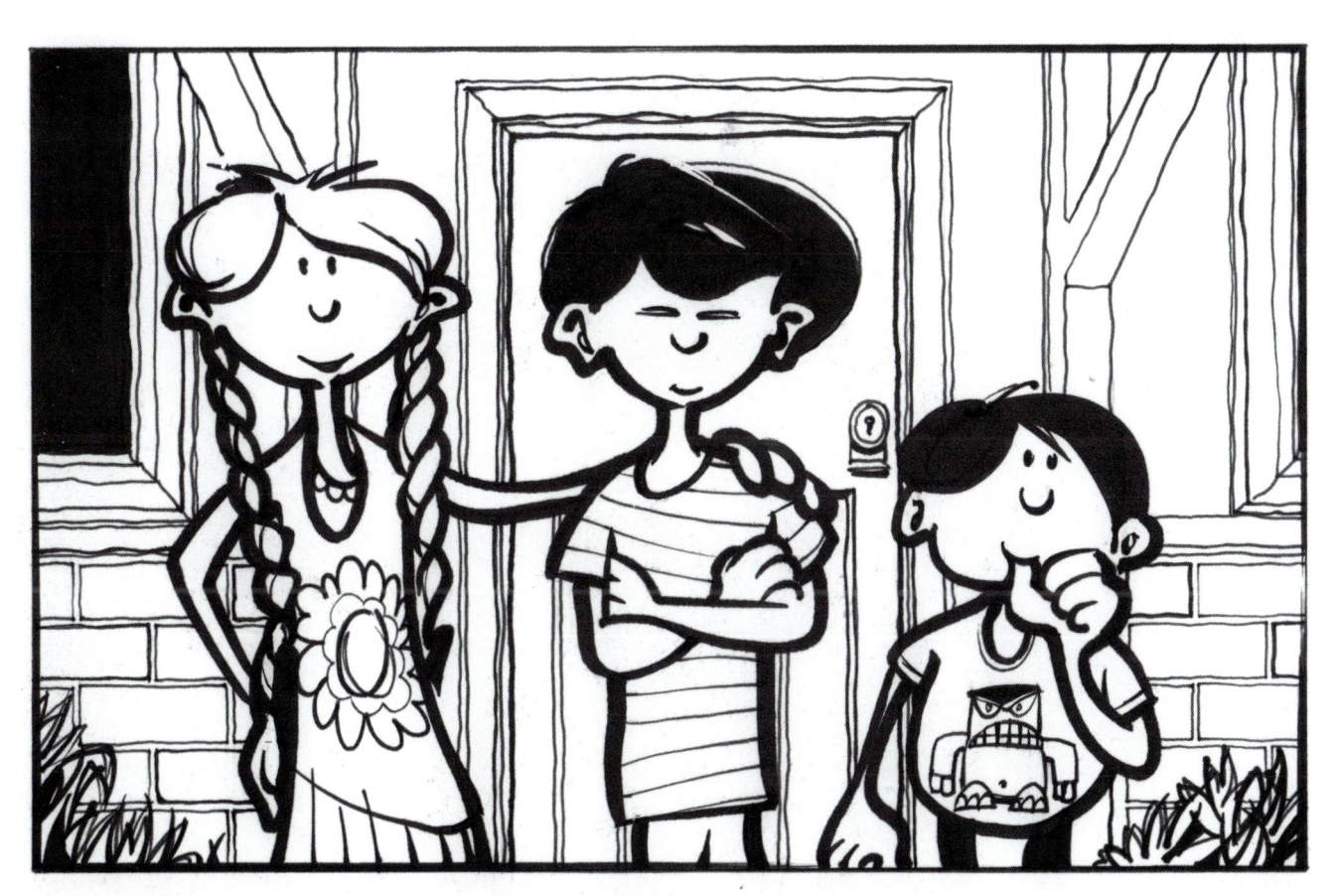

Talking together about an autism diagnosis

Talking to classmates and peers

Again, it can be useful for your child's peers to know about their classmate's diagnosis. Where the child does not want other people to know about their diagnosis, some parents have worked with teachers and schools to develop lessons or whole weeks which look at celebrating difference and diversity etc. This can also be useful in colleges and universities.

The National Autistic Society is able to give guidance and tips on how to move forward with this. A worksheet aimed at primary school-aged children and a lesson plan for older children are reproduced at the back of this book (Appendices three and four).

What if your child does not want you to tell other people about the diagnosis?

Sometimes a person with an ASD will say they do not want other people told about their diagnosis. It is important to be sure that your child knows the possible benefits and disadvantages of other people knowing about the diagnosis.

Often people with an ASD may say no to something because that feels the safest thing to do, but they may not be aware of what it is they are saying no to. The very nature of their difficulties means that they can find it hard to know some of the outcomes of telling other people about their diagnosis. It is therefore not an informed decision unless work has been done to ensure that they understand the possible benefits and possible disadvantages of disclosure.

Try writing things down and talking through the potential benefits as well as the potential difficulties, but be careful not to make promises. Draw up a list of people and discuss together who should be told and who should not be told. Talk about what they would be happy for you to say, and what they would not want you to say.

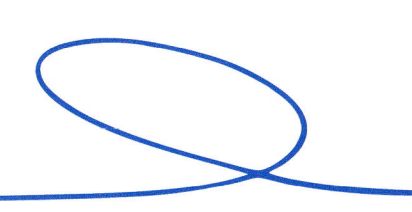

Talking about their diagnosis to adults with an ASD

'I was diagnosed with Asperger syndrome at 30. After this I at least had an identity to relate to. Before then I just thought I was a freak and was totally different from the few friends I had or my family.'
(Taken from *Growing up undiagnosed* by Steve an adult with autism, NAS website, www.autism.org.uk).

Some people do not get a diagnosis until they are in their late adolescence or even well into adulthood. Obviously talking to an adult about their diagnosis will need a very different approach.

Tony Attwood has written a useful chapter on 'Diagnosis in adulthood' in the book *Coming out Asperger* (Murray, D. 2006). He discusses some of the issues and the possible reactions and says that, in his experience, most adults react positively to getting a diagnosis, but there can be a mix of emotions in having received the diagnosis so late in life.

Attwood explains the diagnosis to adults with an 'attributes activity' (p43), where the people in the adult's life spend time talking about the individual's positive qualities and then some of the difficulties they experience, making sure that their positive qualities outweigh the difficulties. At the end of this exercise he explains the difficulties in terms of 'Asperger syndrome' but ensures that the individual comes away with a positive message. He goes on to talk about using the term 'discovery' of Asperger syndrome rather than the term 'diagnosis'. See Useful resources P46.

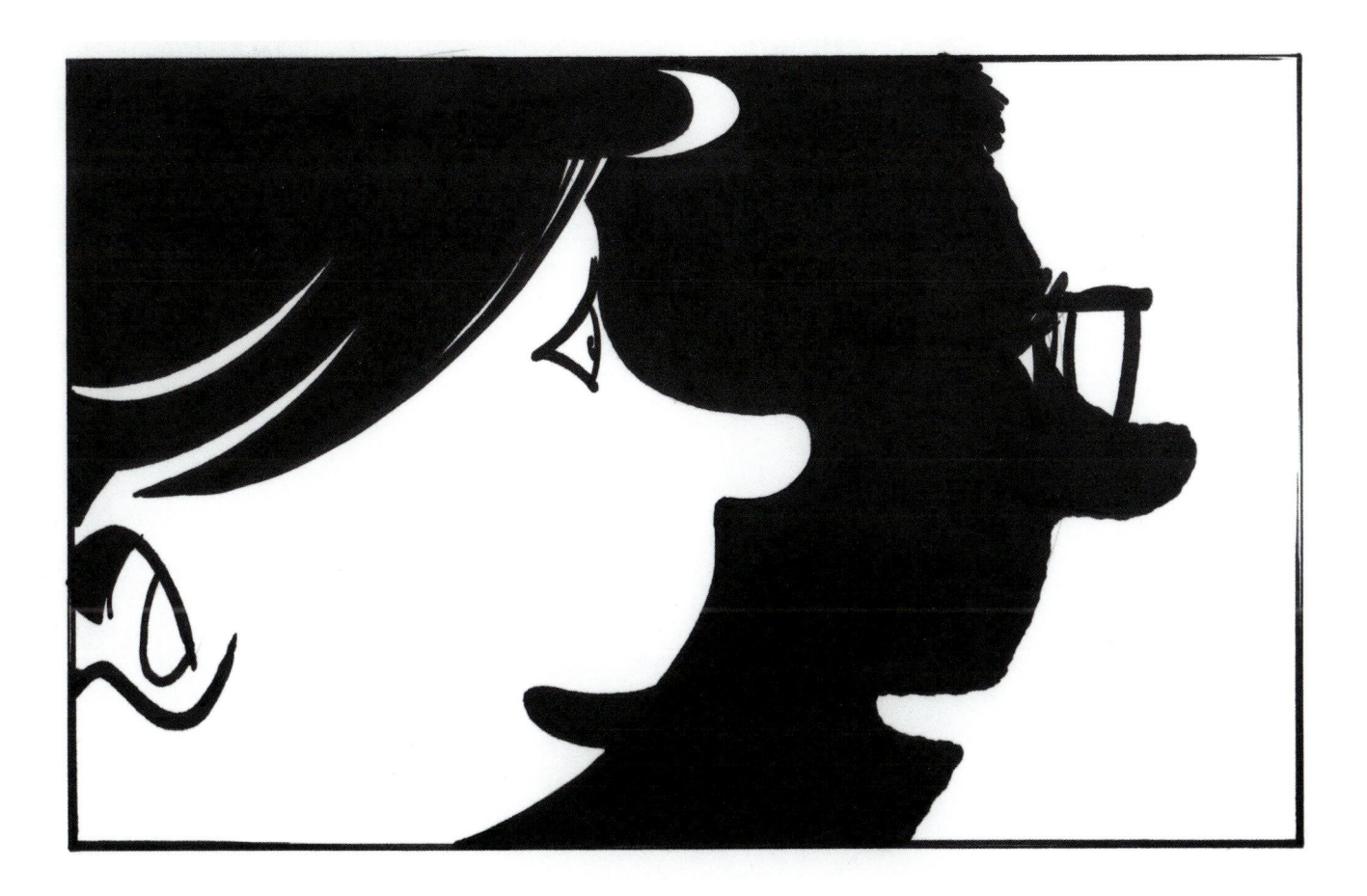

Talking together about an autism diagnosis

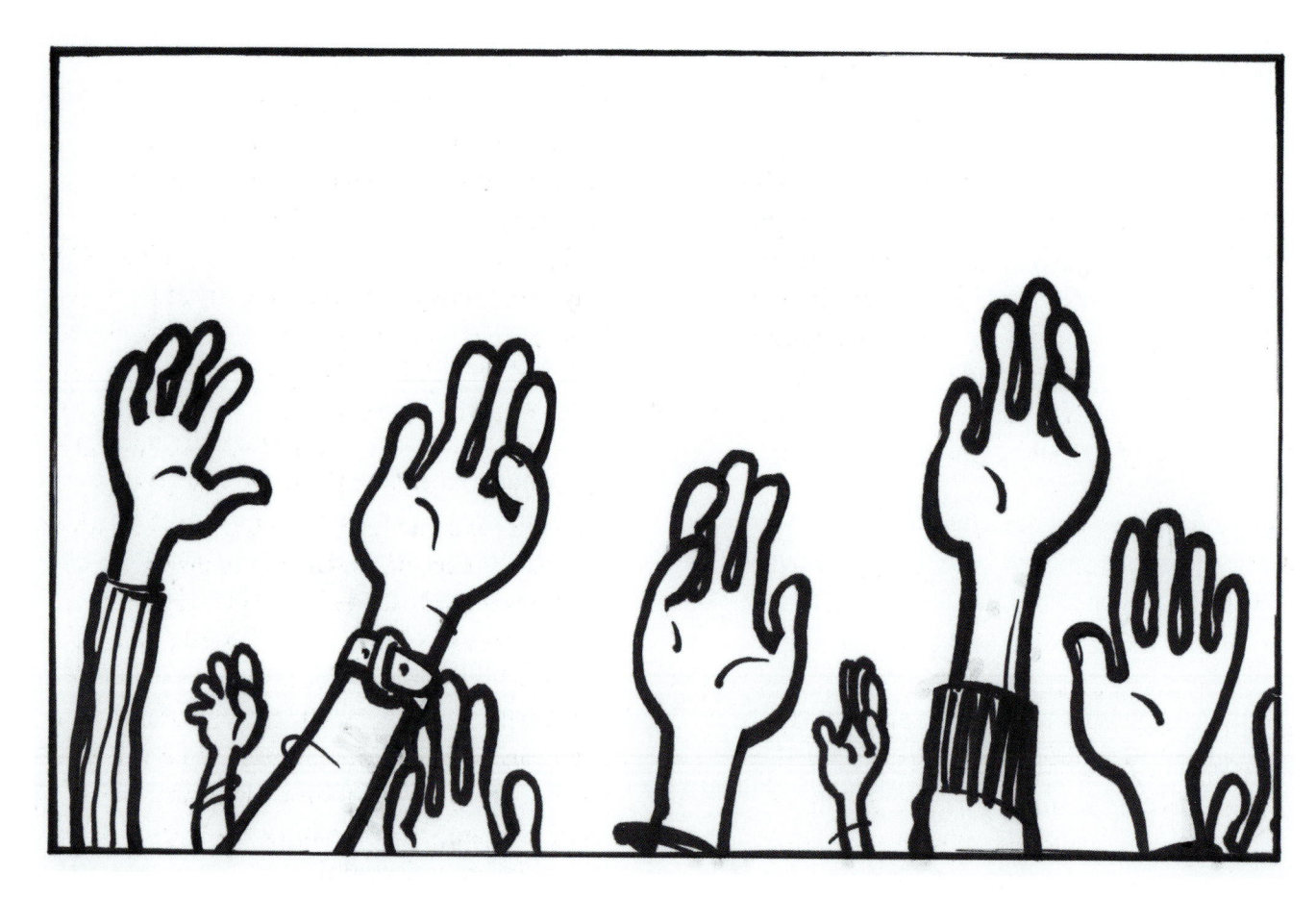

Frequently asked questions
What is an ASD?

How you explain and ASD to your child will vary according to their age and ability. It is very useful to have one or two of the books listed in Useful resources on hand to help with this, as different books will be aimed at different ages and abilities. There are more books being written and published all the time, so it is worth looking at the NAS website to see if there are any new ones that could be helpful (www.autism.org.uk/pubs).

There are several things to bear in mind.

> People with an ASD will be very different from each other but they will also have some things in common. How an ASD affects each person varies greatly.

> The three main areas of difficulty which are common to people with an ASD are:

  > aspects of social communication
  > social relationships
  > social imagination and flexibility of thought.

But there are also other aspects to ASDs that may affect your child, in particular:

> sensory processing difficulties
> difficulties in managing change
> an intense special interest, eg in Harry Potter books.

Be clear about how an ASD affects your child and think of examples to illustrate your conversation.

Explaining difficulties with communication

"You are very good at talking about… , eg Harry Potter, and you are good at telling mummy if you don't want to do something. But you can find it hard to know the right words to say to your teacher and sometimes you don't understand that mummy is only joking when she says, 'my feet are killing me'. Other people with an ASD can find these things hard too. They may not understand what people mean by the words they use."

Explaining social relationships

"Sometimes you prefer to play on your own and at other times you would like to play with the other children at playtime. But you find it hard to know how to play the games and what you need to do. This is part of having an ASD. There are lots of other people with an ASD who find it hard to know how to join in with games and would like to have more friends but don't know how to make friends."

Explaining ASDs generally

"An ASD is something that you can't see. It affects the way your brain works. Everybody with an ASD is different but there are some things that you have in common with other people with an ASD. Some people with an ASD say they find it hard to make sense of the world and often say that they don't know how to act when they are with other people. They can find it hard to know how to talk to other people or to know how to listen, and they can also find it hard to know what other people are thinking and feeling. Some people with an ASD say that they experience life differently to other people. But people with an ASD are also very good at lots of things and you are very good at lots of things. For example you are good at … *[list lots of things]*…. This is partly because of having an ASD and partly because of who you are. We love you very much. Now that we know that you have an ASD we will try to help you with the things you find difficult."

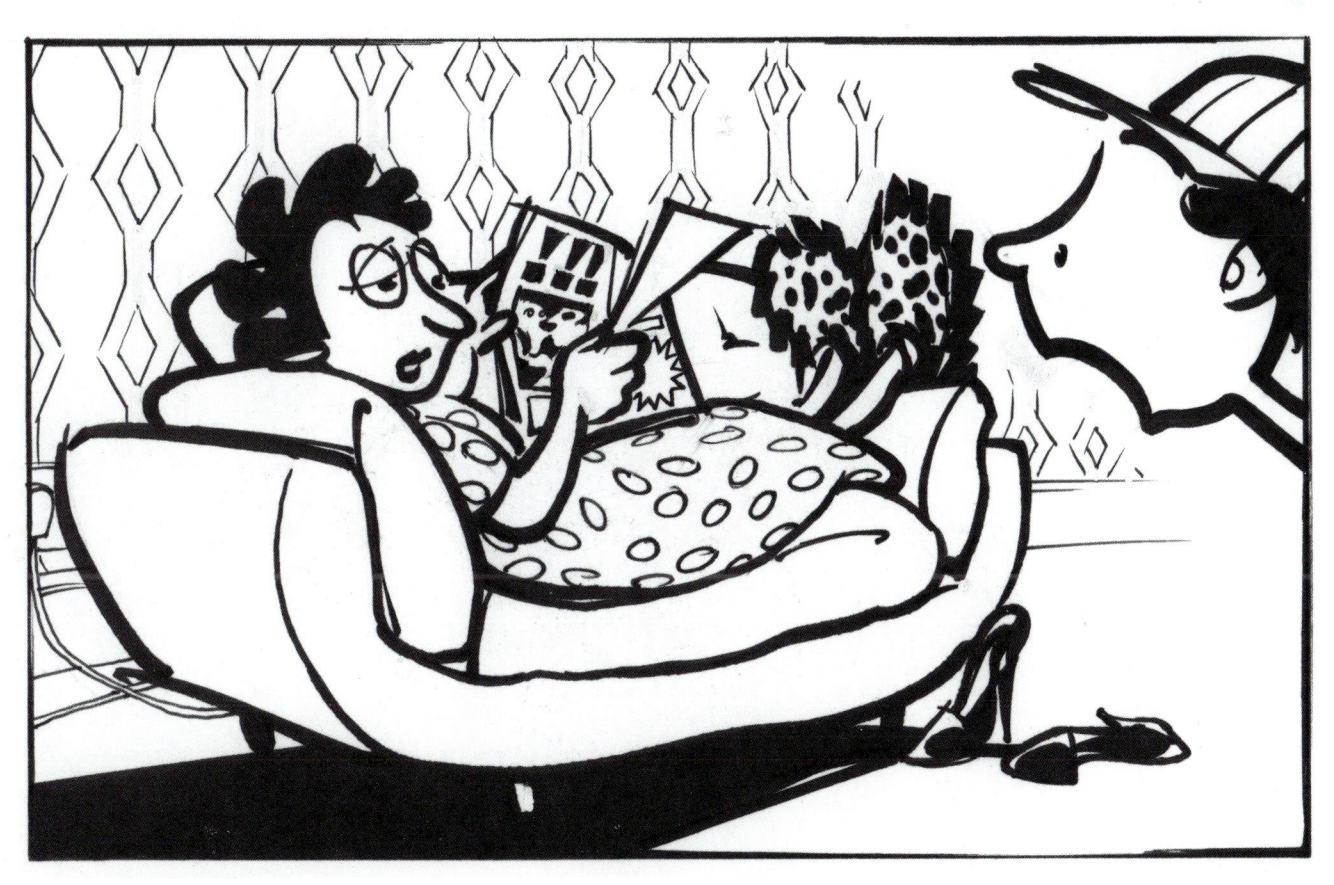

Talking together about an autism diagnosis

How did I get an ASD?

This is a difficult question to answer as we still don't know the exact answer. It might be easiest to be honest and admit that we don't really know. You can talk about some of the current thinking, for example:

> "People are still trying to find out what causes ASDs. It might be that there are several things which can cause ASDs. In some families, several people have ASDs. Scientists are trying to work out why this is. They are looking at people's genes as these may cause ASDs. The important thing to know is that it is not your fault that you have an ASD."
>
> www.kidshealth.org has more information about genes in simple language for children.

Will I always have and ASD?

People with an ASD do not grow out of it so yes, the person will always have an ASD. However, lots of people with an ASD find things a bit easier as they get older and learn how to act in social situations.

You can say to your child that now that you know about their ASD, you can make sure that they gets help with the things that they find difficult. You can help them to know how to act in certain situations and how to let someone know if they are feeling anxious. You can talk about some of the people with an ASD who have achieved great things and who haven't been held back because of it. Finish by reminding your child of their strengths and abilities.

Will I die from an ASD?

No!

Have my brothers and sisters got an ASD?

Some families will have other members with an ASD. Some will have brothers and sisters with some of the characteristics but not enough for a diagnosis, while other family members will have other diagnoses such as attention deficit hyperactivity disorder (ADHD) or dyspraxia. Other families will have children with none of these diagnoses or differences. But every family member will have their own unique range of skills, talents, interests and things they need extra support or help with and that is the important message. As mentioned earlier, you could draw up a list of each family member's skills and areas of difficulty to illustrate this.

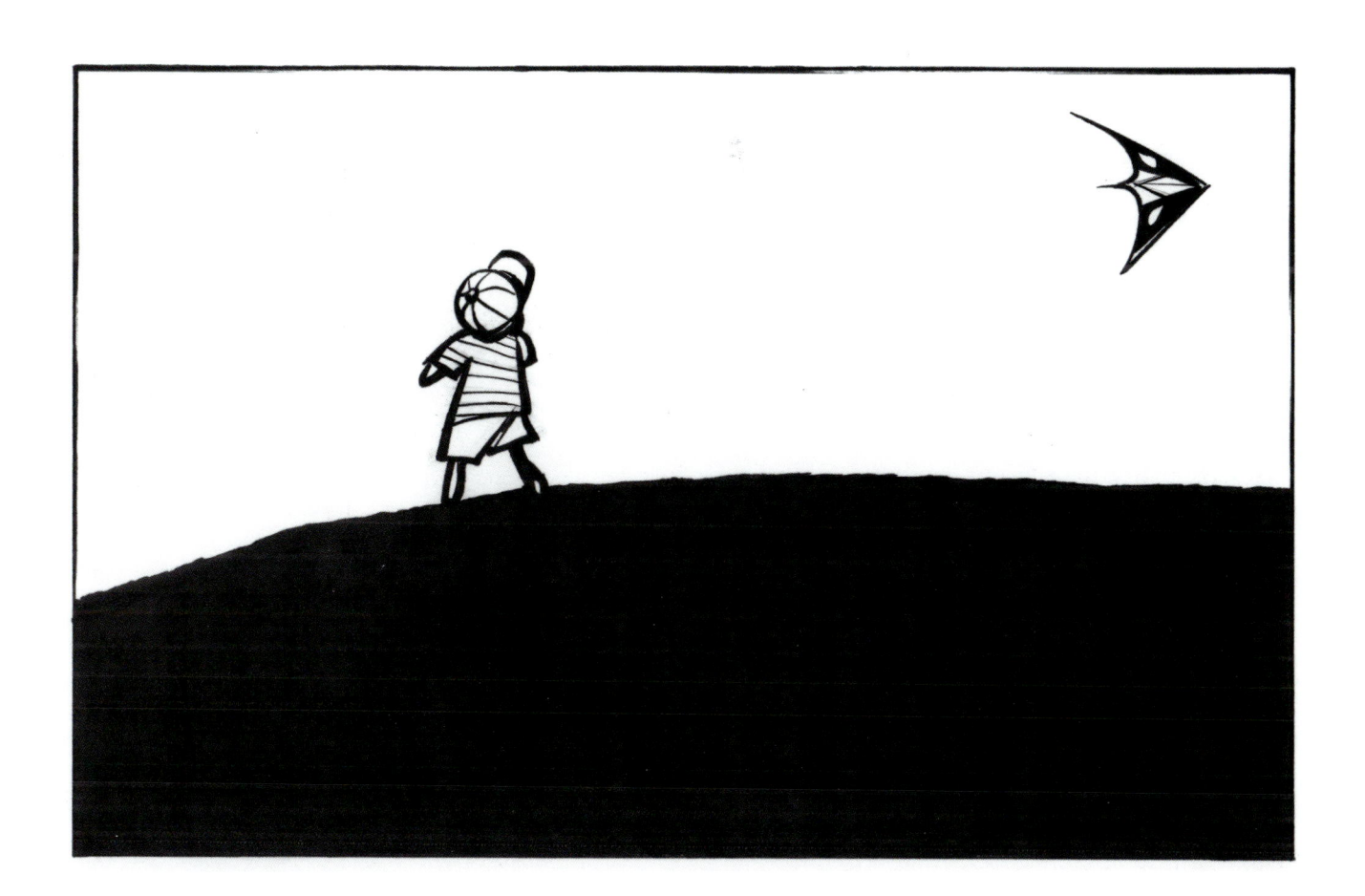

Conclusion

Every person with an ASD is an individual and how an ASD affects each individual will vary hugely. This means that there is often no right or wrong time to talk to your child about having an ASD and there is no one way do it.

It is generally agreed that it is beneficial for children and young people to know about their diagnosis, in a way that is meaningful for them, sooner rather than later. It should not be something that they feel unable to speak about and the initial discussion is the start of the process, not the end. Where possible, it is best to talk about differences rather than difficulties and it is particularly important to reassure your child that their particular skills and strengths are valued and respected.

Talking together about an autism diagnosis

Appendix 1 – Explaining an autism diagnosis

Example for a person with learning difficulties

This is me. My name is Alex.

I am years old

I like

_____

_____

I don't like

_____

_____

I have autism

It means that I need help with some things

Some things I need help with are:

_____

_____

_____

_____

It also means I am good at some things

Some things that I am good at are:

_____

_____

_____

_____

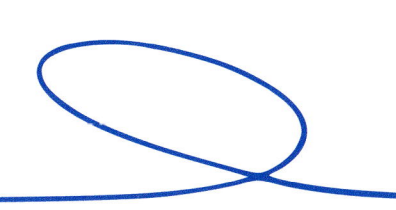

Appendix 2

Making a *Pictures of me* workbook

Introduction

Explaining an ASD to a person with autism or Asperger syndrome is far from easy. An ASD is an extremely complex disorder and very difficult to explain to most people, let alone someone who actually has it. Carol Gray, consultant to students with ASDs, has designed *Pictures of me*, a Social Story™ designed to introduce an individual with Asperger syndrome or high-functioning autism to their personality, talent and diagnosis. Here we reproduce the Social Story which can be adapted to suit the specific needs of each individual.

This article first appeared in the autumn 1996 issue of *The Morning News* pp1-14 and is reproduced with kind permission of Carol Gray.

Pictures of me – introducing students with an ASD to their talents, personality and diagnosis

By Carol Gray

Pictures of me is a special Social Story™. Following a 'workbook' style format, *Pictures of me* offers a series of activities designed to introduce a student with Asperger syndrome to his personality, talents and diagnosis. To date, *Pictures of me* has been piloted with upper elementary age students. *Pictures of me* uses aspects of both Social Stories (Gray & Garand 1993) and Comic Strip Conversations™ (Gray, 1994) to assist parents and professionals in sharing diagnostic and personal information with a student.

The Social Story is modified to meet the unique and specific needs of each student. Activities directed by the story include the completion of three lists and several stories. The result is a process of positive self discovery. The completed workbook is a resource that provides a student with a 'souvenir' of himself, a tangible reference containing important personal information.

Pictures of me was initiated by Phil and Kathi Hunt, whose 10 year old son, Joel, had recently been diagnosed with Asperger syndrome. Phil and Kathi asked for assistance in explaining the diagnosis to Joel in a way that would be meaningful for him and easy to understand. The result was *Pictures of me*, first piloted with the Hunts early in 1996. The author expresses sincere appreciation to the Hunts for their permission to share Joel's completed workbook as a sample in this article.

Pictures of me is reviewed by the parents prior to meeting with the child so that the story may be revised and individualised for the student. Creative additions to the story can improve its effectiveness. For example, parents may choose to add personalised explanations to the story.

In addition, modifications may need to be made to ensure that the story accurately describes a student's family, for example, in cases of divorce, single parent families or foster families. This article and sample *Pictures of me* Social Story share a diagnosis of Asperger syndrome. With minor modifications the Social Story could be tailored for students with high-functioning autism as well.

Completing *Pictures of me* requires a relaxed and quiet environment. The workbook takes up to two hours to complete and may require a few break sessions.

A time of day that is likely to be free of interruptions, for example, early evening at an office or school, or during the day at the student's home, is suggested. The student is encouraged to select a favourite activity and treat that can be shared during break times. Phil, Kathi and Joel Hunt met with this author in an office at Jenison High School.

Talking together about an autism diagnosis

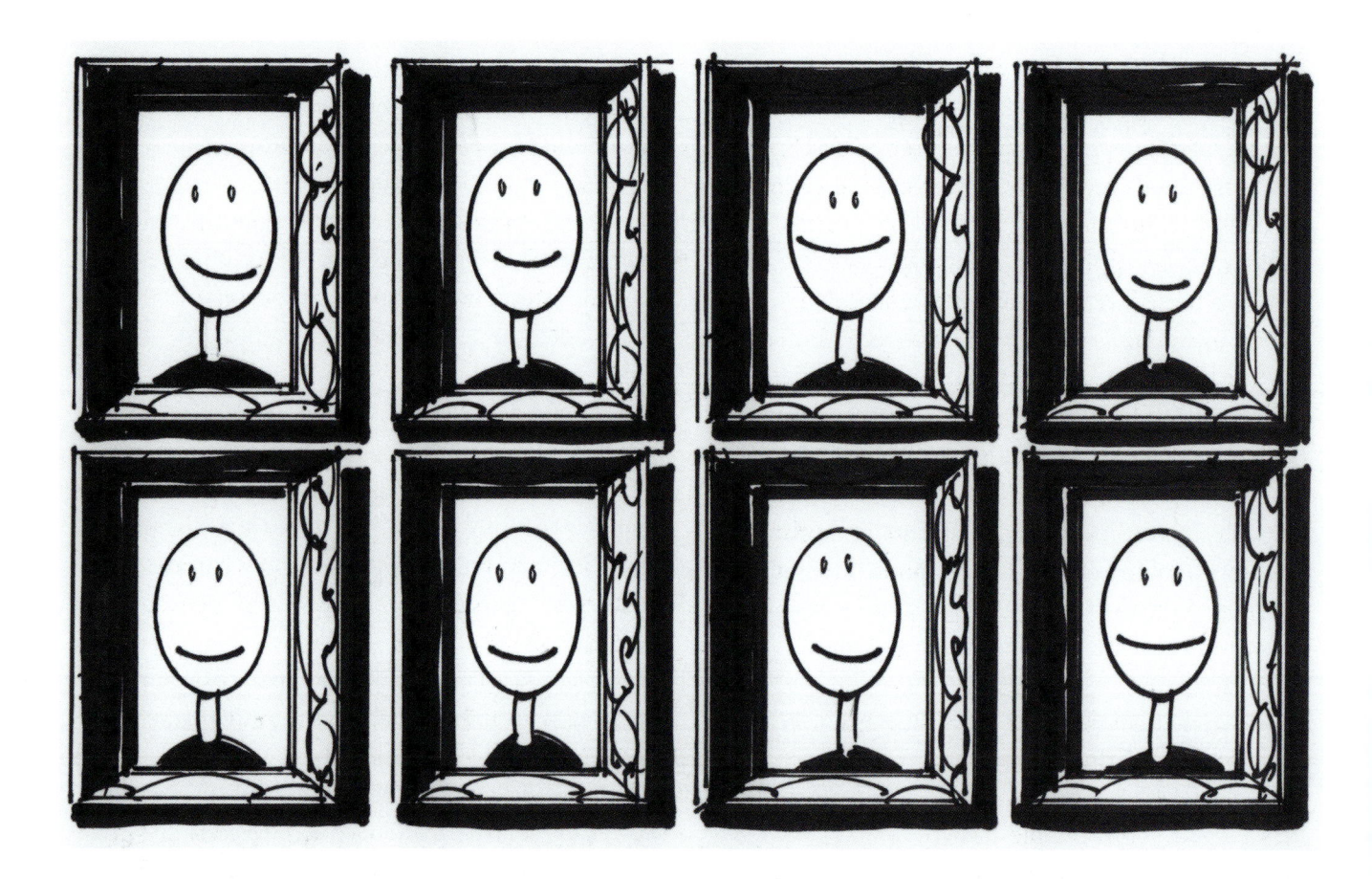

The *Pictures of Me* Social Story

The title page As mentioned earlier, the *Pictures of me* Social Story directs the activities of the participants. *Pictures of me* opens with a title page that introduces the student and those who will be helping complete the workbook.

Page 1 The first page of the story contains two large, side by side, blank vertical boxes. These are frames for pictures that are drawn by the parents. Under these frames, are titles for the pictures that will be drawn in the frames. For the Hunts the frames were titled *My son Joel by Mrs Hunt* and *My son Joel by Mr Hunt*. This page is often assigned as homework for the parents to be completed at another time. This usually is not a problem: students often enjoy seeing homework assigned to their parents! Directions for completion of these first drawings by the parents are included in the opening text.

Page 2 This author believes it is important to attribute personal traits to personality and talent to keep Asperger syndrome in perspective. In general, attributing personal traits first to personality, personal preference or a student's age may be a helpful rule of thumb. A student's disability ends up playing a smaller role when it is perceived as one of several factors that may explain a given trait or behaviour (Gray, 1996).

The second page introduces a student to his personality and talents within the completion of two lists. These lists are completed with everyone working together. The student decides who will serve as 'secretary'. In this case, Joel volunteered to record the lists of his personality traits and talents.

Pages 3, 4, 5 and 6 The next four pages of the workbook require each person to draw a picture of the student's personality and talents.

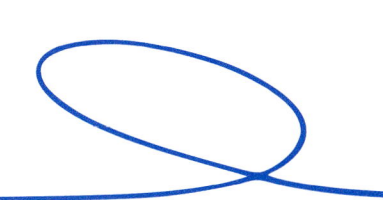

After these pictures were drawn, they are shared with the other *Pictures of me* participants. Each person has the opportunity to describe their drawing and to explain why they needed to include certain items in their picture. Joel had a real strength in his ability to read and this author drew Joel playing *Nintendo*, illustrating his skill at mastering video games. Joel's father used his son's picture and talents as an opportunity to draw Joel as a hero. Mr Hunt's picture illustrated how Joel had saved the life of Lexi, Joel's sister, who had swallowed some pennies. In sharing his picture with the other participants, Mr Hunt proudly shared his gratitude for Joel's quick action and heroism.

Page 7 The seventh page of the workbook introduces the student to his diagnosis. Part of that introduction includes a reference to *The Morning News Pen Pal Registry** (Gray, 1995). The registry was developed for people with an ASD as a continually expanding resource meeting others who share similar interests and experiences. Mentioning the Pen Pal registry in the story directs the student to others who share the same diagnosis. The registry provides tangible evidence of other people with Asperger syndrome: their ages, addresses, interests and in many cases photos.

Recognising the individual nature of the disorder, the description of Asperger syndrome is presented as a list that is completed by the participants. This is a list of skills that may be more difficult because of Asperger syndrome, although mention is also made of positive aspects of the disorder (Attwood, T. 1998). Other information on Asperger syndrome is available to the student through the parents, and/or subsequent meetings with the professional.

Page 8 On the last page of the story the student is reminded of his support system: the people who will continue to assist the student in the future and how they will help. Applying theory of mind information (Baron-Cohen, S. 1995), this page explains what adults know, mentioning who has information about Asperger syndrome and growing up and how that information can be accessed. In addition, the feelings the parents and professionals have for the student are expressed in writing. Mrs Anderson, mentioned on this page, is Joel's speech therapist.

Pictures of me defines the starting point for a gradual process of self discovery that requires continuing guidance and assistance from parents and professionals. The *Pictures of me* Social Story, workbook, and activities are only a beginning. Follow up activities are currently being developed. In the meantime, parents and professionals are encouraged to provide opportunities for questions and discussions as a student considers and applies personal information.

In summary, *Pictures of me* is a Social Story that guides a series of workbook style activities. The goal is to successfully introduce a student to his diagnosis, personality and talents. Activities are completed by the student, parents and a professional, and involve the collective completion of lists and drawings. The end result is an individualised, illustrated Social Story that introduces a student to his diagnosis, while at the same time keeping that information in perspective among other positive personality traits and talents.

Pictures of me – a book about a great person

By Joel Hunt

With illustrations by
Mrs Hunt
Mr Hunt
Joel Hunt
Mrs Gray

I have a personality

All people have personalities. On the inside, I have a personality. Personality can be a hard thing to explain. I have a wonderful personality. My mom, my dad, Mrs Gray, and I tried to think of words to describe my personality.
Here is our list:

1. I like Yoshi
2. Friendly
3. Good brother
4. Weather
5. Happy
6. Fun
7. Out going
8. Nice
9. Enthusiastic

I have talent

All people have talents. On the inside I have talent. Talents are a little easier to explain than personalities. Some people can draw great pictures. Some people have wonderful memories, or school work is very easy for them. I have talents too. My mom, dad, Mrs Gray and I tried to think of words to describe my talents. Here is our list:

1. Intelligent
2. Actor
3. Nintendo player
4. Imagination
5. _____
6. _____

My name is Joel. I am a wonderful person. Many people think I'm pretty neat, including my mom and dad. Above, they have drawn their pictures of me. Mom drew the one on the left, dad drew the picture on the right. This is how they think I look on the outside

This is my Mom's picture of me on the inside. Here you see my personality and talents. It's a work of art. She signed her name to it, just like a great artist.

This is my Dad's picture of me on the inside. Here you see my personality and talents. It's a work of art. He signed his name to it just like a great artist.

This is my picture of me on the inside. Here you see my personality and talents. It's a work of art. I signed my name to it just like a great artist.

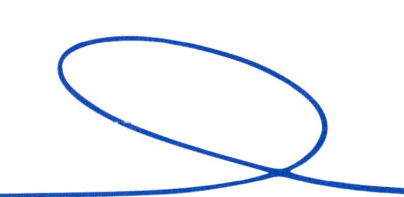

This is a complete picture of me on the inside. I have drawn pictures my personality, my talents, my interests, my likes and dislikes, and my Asperger syndrome. I have signed my name to my drawing like a great artist.

33

Talking together about an autism diagnosis

My mom and dad love me very much. They can help me develop my wonderful personality. They will help me develop my talents and interests.

They can also help me with the things that are more difficult for me. Some of the things that are difficult for me will be difficult because I am growing up. All people have some difficult times growing up.

They can also help me with the things that are difficult for me because of Asperger syndrome. Mrs Gray, Mrs Anderson and my teachers will help me too. They know how to help me learn to develop my personality and my talents. They know about Asperger syndrome too.

I might have questions about Asperger syndrome. That's where Mrs Gray will help me. She knows all about students and growing up. She was once a student, and she grew up and she knows it is sometimes difficult and sometimes easy. She also knows about Asperger syndrome. Whenever my parents or I have questions about Asperger syndrome, we can ask Mrs Gray.

Mrs Gray likes me very much. She thinks I have a great personality and a lot of talent. She feels very lucky to know me.

I have Asperger syndrome

Some people have Asperger syndrome. Many of the students in the Pen Pal registry have Asperger syndrome just like I do. Asperger syndrome can be a difficult thing to explain. I cannot see Asperger syndrome, but I know it's there. Asperger syndrome may make some things more difficult for me than for other students.

On the inside I have Asperger syndrome. Asperger syndrome can be a hard thing to explain. My mom, my dad, Mrs Gray and I tried to list things that may be more difficult for me because of my Asperger syndrome.

Here is our list:

1. Looking at people

2. Staying on subject

3. Making friends

4. Understanding others

5. _____

6. _____

7. _____

8. _____

All people have difficulty with these things as they grow up. I may have more difficulty with these things than most people because I have Asperger syndrome.

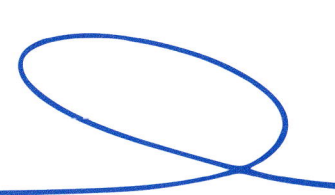

Appendix 3 NAS autism worksheet for primary school aged children

Name:

Hello, my name is Ziggy. I am here to tell you about your new classmate who has something called autism. Write their name below.

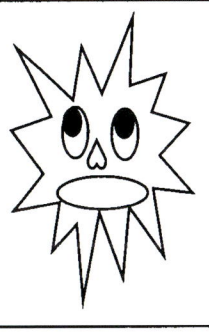

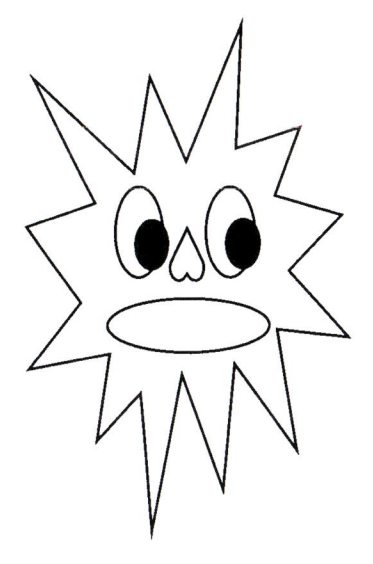

We are all good at some things but not so good at others. In the boxes below, write or draw some things you are good at. In the other box, write or draw things you find difficult.

I am good at:	I am not so good at:

35

Talking together about an autism diagnosis

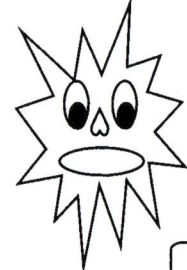

If a person uses a wheelchair, you know they have difficulty walking. If someone is blind, you know they cannot see. These people have disabilities. Autism is a special kind of disability.

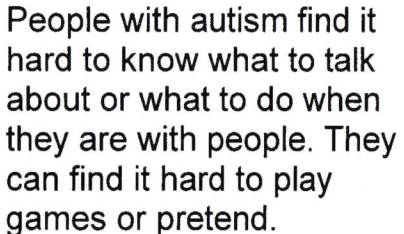

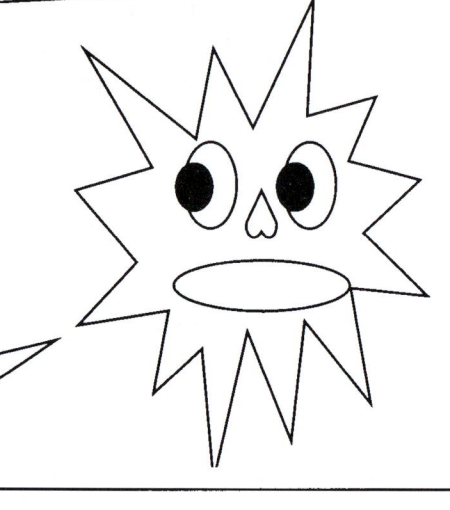

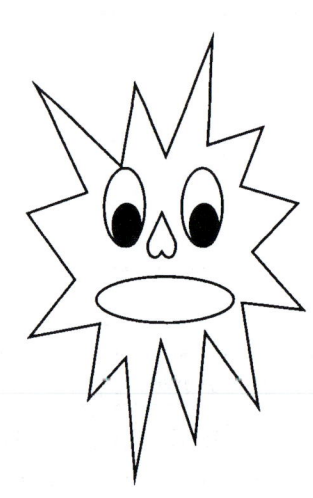

People with autism find it hard to know what to talk about or what to do when they are with people. They can find it hard to play games or pretend.

You may find your new classmate does not talk in the same way as you. They may say very little or repeat what you say. They do not mean to be rude or tease you.

They may talk over and over about the same thing, like dinosaurs. Try telling them they can only talk about this thing they are really interested in at certain times, such as playtime. You may need to keep reminding them of this rule.

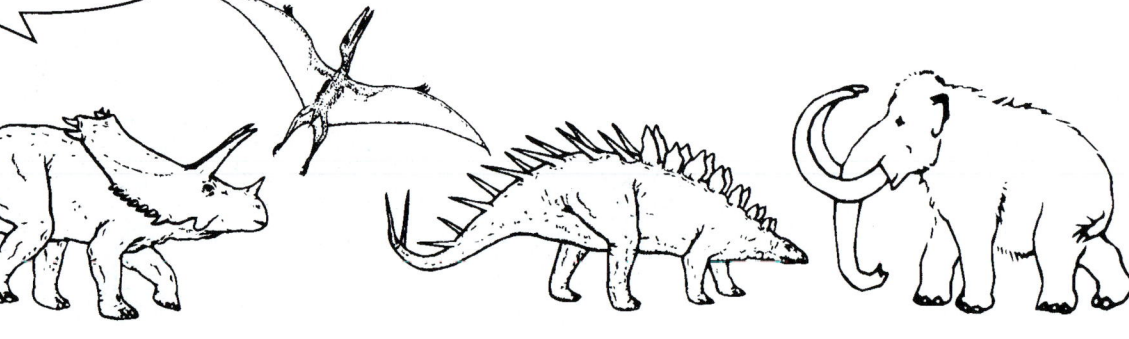

Colour us in

36

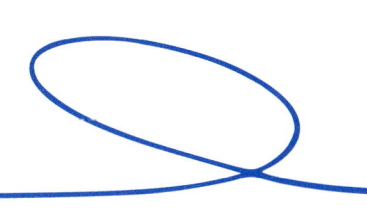

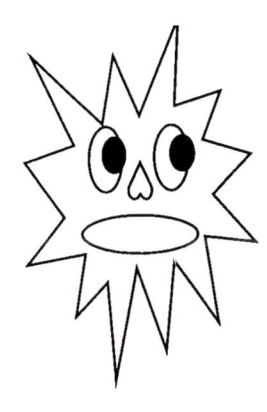

Sometimes you might find it is difficult to tell when someone is joking with you or teasing you. People with autism find this extra hard and you might have to tell them 'That was a joke' or 'I was only joking'.

Can you tell what the following faces are trying to express? Write your answers on the dotted lines. I have done the first one for you.

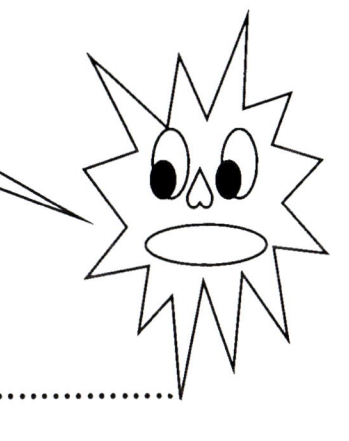

I'm happy ....　　　..............................

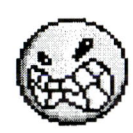

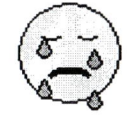

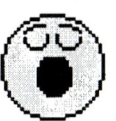

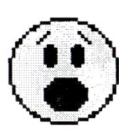

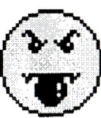

....　　　..............................

....　　　..............................

People with autism find understanding faces very difficult. Sometimes when you smile at someone with autism, they might not smile back. This does not mean they are being rude or don't want to be friendly. They just find it difficult to understand that you want to be their friend and you might need to tell them that.

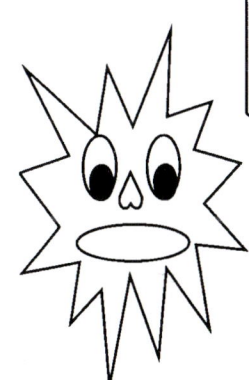

I am your friend

37

Talking together about an autism diagnosis

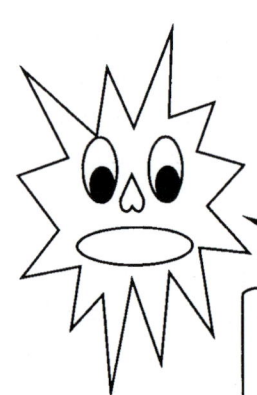

> When you were very small, you had to learn to be polite like saying "please" and "thank you". You also had to learn not to point at someone and say "You are really fat".

> Rules like these are really difficult to learn if you have autism. If someone with autism says something like that, they don't mean to be rude. It's not telling tales if you ask your teacher to explain to them that what they are saying is rude and why they shouldn't say it.

> All children sometimes behave in ways that seem naughty. It is really hard to understand but children with autism don't know when they are being naughty. Your teacher may have to explain to them something is wrong.

> Children with autism also find it difficult to play your games. If you are playing a game with your friends, someone with autism might find it more fun to sit or play by themselves. You or your teacher may have to keep showing them how to play your games and how much fun it can be. It may help if you explain the rules every time you play.

> Please talk to your teacher if there is anything you don't understand in this worksheet. I hope you will enjoy making friends with your new classmate. Goodbye for now.
>
> **Ziggy**

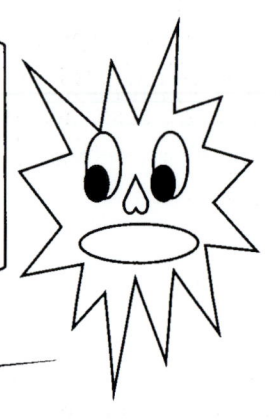

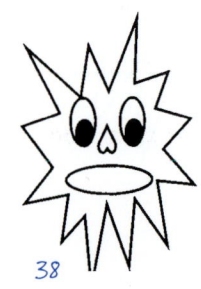

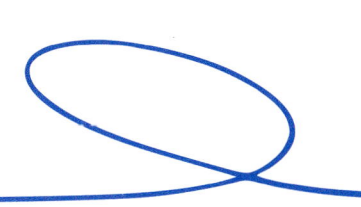

Appendix 4

The National Autistic Society school lesson plan

Introduction and plan

These materials have been prepared for a two-lesson introduction to ASDs They include two case study sheets and some games for introducing ASDs to a class.

Points to highlight in the lessons are:

> an ASD affects a person's social and communication skills
> ASDs are a broad spectrum of need and different individuals have different needs
> structure can really help someone with an ASD
> it is important to treat all people with an ASD as individuals.

■ Lesson 1

1 – 10 mins

Do a 10-minute brainstorm with the whole class on what social and communication skills mean:

> speaking
> listening
> making friends
> understanding people.

This list can be added to.

You can also use the ideas game on pages 40 – 41

10 – 30 mins

Explain that autism is a disability that affects a person's social and communication skills and that it affects different people in different ways. Over the next two lessons the class will be looking at what it involves, how it can affect different people and discussing what support can help people with an ASD, leading to a written piece on the subject.

- Hand out case study sheets including questions.

Read through with the class and have a discussion. Ask the students to study the different ways David and Helen are supported in matters of structure, routine and anxiety then ask them to answer the questions below:

> how does an ASD affect David and Helen?
> how independently do you think each person is able to live? (Give three reasons for your answers)
> how would David and Helen deal with social situations?
> in what ways are David and Helen able to communicate and express themselves?

30 – 55 mins

In groups of four or five ask students to discuss these questions. Give each of the groups a case study to work on and ask them to answer the question below:

> how can you best support someone with an ASD?

Ask them to prepare three key points for a class discussion on the issue in the next lesson.

55 – 60 mins

Plenary – draw class back together and go over the key points discussed in the lesson.

■ Lesson 2

1 – 10 mins

Recap points from previous lesson. What is an ASD?

10 – 25 mins

Go back into groups and go over key points discussed last lesson, for whole class discussion.

25 – 50 mins

Class discussion on how to best support someone with an ASD.

39

Talking together about an autism diagnosis

Draw out points such as being reliable, making things structured, giving clear instructions and helping individuals not to feel anxious. Sign language can help for those who are non-verbal. Emphasise that both case studies are very different but David Downes is very able: but Helen Burnell is much more dependent. Highlight the importance of treating people as individuals with different needs.

If a person with an ASD is in the class, they should be encouraged to explain things that help them. Other students should be encouraged to explain things they do that help support that person.

Games for introducing ASDs to a class

Memorise a sequence game

This is a game that some people with an ASD who have a fascination with order and sequences would find very enjoyable and would be very good at.

Ask the class to form a circle and choose one person to start the game by saying, 'Today I went to the shop and brought myself a...', thinking of an item and adding it to the end of a sentence. The next person in the circle then has to say the sentence with the item the last person said along with their own choice of item. This continues around the circle until someone makes a mistake. That person is then asked to sit down, and the game continues around and around the circle until the last person is left. You can adapt the sentence to suit the class' interest.

> - You can introduce an off-putting noise such as a drum, vacuum cleaner or a radio. This will make it harder for people to concentrate, giving a clearer understanding of why people with an ASD find distractions hard to cope with.
> - Ask the students how this game made them feel. Did any of them feel frustrated when the loud noise started?

Sensory game

This game is good for helping students to understand why unexpected occurrences can be uncomfortable, a difficulty which many people with an ASD have to cope with every day.

Select a range of edible and textured objects and place them in a box. These things can range from instant coffee granules to jelly. Ask for one volunteer to sit up at the front of the class and blindfold them. With each of your selected sensory objects, allow the student to either taste or feel them. The more unexpected the sensory object, the more surprised the student will feel. Things like coffee granules will be very unpleasant and give a better understanding of how unexpected events can sometimes be distressing. Ask for some other volunteers to have a go at this task. Ask them to explain how they felt when they experienced a taste or feel of an object they did not like.

You could also offer the class something to eat or drink that looks like something they are used to but in fact is something else like a chocolate spread sandwich, with a dollop of mustard hidden inside or a glass of lemonade or water with some colourless flavouring such as aniseed. The unexpected can be more shocking than we expect. Finally, ask them how important trust and respect are when building relationships with people with an ASD.

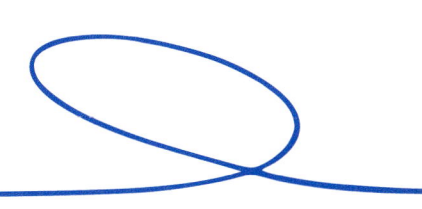

Speaking game

Address the class in a severe tone of voice but use friendly, positive words. Then speak to them in a friendly voice, but using negative words eg 'you are a very naughty group and I am angry with you all.'

This highlights the importance of tone and volume in communication.

People with an ASD can miss these clues.

Listening and understanding game

Address the class in 'gibberish' or a foreign language, at the same time focusing on one pupil. Through gesture, indicate that you wish them to stand. When they do so, ask them why they are standing. Tell them you weren't indicating for them to stand but were actually indicating to them to do something else – dependent upon what your gesture looked like!

This highlights the importance of non-verbal clues in language and how we react to them instinctively.

Explain that someone with an ASD would not be able to follow non-verbal clues. They might misinterpret them or not notice them at all.

Making friends game

One young person with Asperger syndrome, Mark Segar, put together a list of his 'rules for life' – advice and tips for others with Asperger syndrome and autism on how to interact and communicate with people. Share the following examples with the class:

> if you wish to talk to someone, the best thing to do when you first meet them is just to talk to them and NOT get too close
> suitable boundaries may vary from one person to another
> it is important not to appear too eager
> if you are a man, don't wear too much after-shave
> don't talk to just anyone, make sure it's someone you like.

Ask the class:

> what do you do when you go out?
> do you go with someone?
> how do you get a girlfriend or boyfriend?

What do the class think it would be like doing these things for someone who doesn't understand the ways that people communicate and interact?

Personal space game

Make two pupils face each other at a space of about five metres apart. Ask one to walk towards the other and stop when it's comfortable. Ask them why they feel it's comfortable.

Then tell them to take one more step, then another, until they are practically touching.

> Ask the class where this level of closeness is acceptable – eg on the bus, in a football crowd, on the tube etc.
> Ask them where it is not acceptable – eg at the beach
> Ask how they know about this understanding, eg are the rules written down?

Highlight that we do things instinctively, but people with an ASD have to learn these social rules which are changing all the time, dependent upon who is involved, where and when.

Talking together about an autism diagnosis

Case study 1: David Downes

David Downes is an artist who has Asperger syndrome. He is becoming increasingly well known for his art and works part time in an art shop, supported by The National Autistic Society's employment consultancy, Prospects.

David is very successful in his art work. He completed an MA at the Royal College of Art in Communication Design in 1996. In September 1999, he set out to record the BBC's most important architecture at the turn of the century. In June 2000 he became artist in-residence to BBC Heritage. In 2000 David's life and career featured in a book, *Artists emerging* (Paine, S. and Phillip, T. 2000).

David was diagnosed with Asperger syndrome in July 2002. David has always been aware that he deals with things like money and relationships differently from other people. 90% of the time David says that he feels like he does not have Asperger syndrome. He explains that his disability means he can see things very clearly, like the buildings he paints, but that other thing`s are sometimes confusing, such as communicating with people. David finds unpredictable events difficult to cope with. At an important exhibition that David had this year, he became anxious because an aspect of the show did not go as planned. Because David was anxious, he forgot about other important aspects of the show, even though he had only been working on them the day before.

Before David was diagnosed with Asperger syndrome, he did not understand why he would get so anxious about things. Since he has been diagnosed he and his family can find ways of dealing with problems. David's family have been very supportive throughout his life and have helped him to achieve his full potential.

David found out about Prospects, the NAS employment consultancy that supports people with autism and Asperger syndrome. They helped him to find a job and support him at work. David said that Prospects help him at work by offering different perspectives on a problem and coping strategies with uncomfortable situations. They have given David support and advice when he has organised exhibitions.

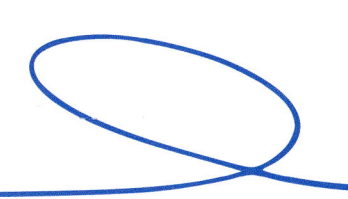

Case Study 1: David Downes – differentiated work sheet

David Downes is an artist who has Asperger syndrome, a disability that affects the way a person understands other people and the world.

David was diagnosed with Asperger syndrome in July 2002.

David says that having Asperger syndrome means he can see things very clearly, such as the buildings he paints, but that other things can be confusing, such as having conversations with people.

David finds unpredictable events difficult to cope with. At an important exhibition David had this year, he became anxious because a part of the show did not go as planned. Because David was anxious, he forgot about other important parts of the show, even though he had only been working on them the day before.

Before David knew he had Asperger syndrome he did not understand why he would get so anxious about things. Now he knows, he can understand his feelings more and he and his family are able to find ways of dealing with problems he may have.

David's family are very supportive and help him a great deal.

Case Study 2: Helen Burnell –

Helen Burnell was diagnosed with autism at the age of five and attended the first National Autistic Society (NAS) School in 1965. Back then there was even less understanding about ASDs and psychiatrists believed that Helen should go to a residential home. It was with the help of her mum, Ilse, that Sybil Elgar, a dedicated teacher, and a group of determined parents that the first NAS school was set up: the Sybil Elgar School for children with autism. Helen was one of ten children who attended the school in Ealing. The school followed the same curriculum as the national system and taught the children, who were deemed unable to be educated, to talk, read, write and socialise with others.

Once Helen and other pupils reached the age of 15, their parents realised that there were no other options or education available to them and worked together to provide a safe, happy environment for their children to grow and develop into adults. They worked together to build a residency in Somerset called Somerset Court, where Helen still lives today.

Helen is one of the less able residents and because of this she is unable to work. This does not mean that she prefers to do nothing. Helen enjoys routine and helps her carers with keeping her home tidy. She also enjoys activities in the form of games which help her with social situations, swimming and going on outings.

Helen uses Makaton, a form of sign language and symbols, to communicate because she is unable to talk. This allows Helen to express herself. Not being able to have any form of communication and expression would be very frustrating and could result in negative behaviour. When Helen was a young child she would often break things as this was the only way she was able to express herself without Makaton.

Talking together about an autism diagnosis

Helen is very attached to her mother and father and, with the help of a residency like Somerset Court, Helen and her family are able to have a positive and loving relationship and she is able to be quite independent.

'Somerset Court has given Helen an environment where she is able to get the most out of life.'
Helen's mum, Ilse Burnell

Case Study 2: Helen Burnell – differentiated work sheet

Helen Burnell was diagnosed with autism when she was five and attended the first National Autistic Society school in 1965.

Helen is unable to talk.

Helen now lives in a residential service in Somerset called Somerset Court.

Helen is one of the less able people at Somerset Court. She is not able to work.

She enjoys routine and helps the people who care for her to keep her home tidy.

Helen enjoys activities like games and playing games can help her to work with other people.

Helen also enjoys swimming and going on outings.

Helen now uses a form of sign language to communicate because she is unable to talk.

Before she leant this sign language she would often get frustrated because she couldn't communicate with people. She often behaved badly because of this.

Helen is very close to her mother and father and with the help of them and the staff at Somerset Court is able to lead a positive life.

Helen's Mum, Ilse Burnell says: *"Somerset Court has given Helen an environment where she is able to get the most out of life.'*

These lesson plans were produced by Jenny Rowbottom, a former teacher and member of the NAS press team, for our make school make sense campaign.

References

*Attwood, T. (1998). *The Asperger's syndrome: a guide for parents and professionals,* London: Jessica Kingsley Publishers

*Attwood, T. (2006). *The complete guide to Asperger's syndrome,* London: Jessica Kingsley Publishers

*Doherty, K., McNally, P. and Sherrard E. (2003). *I have Autism…What's that?* Lisburn: Down Lisburn Trust

**Gillberg, C. (1991). 'Clinical and neurobiological aspects of Asperger syndrome in six family studies.' In U. Frith (ed) *Autism and Asperger syndrome,* Cambridge: Cambridge University Press, p138

*Gray, C. (2002). *My Social Stories book,* London: Jessica Kingsley Publishers

*Jackson, J. (2002) p120 – *Multicoloured mayhem,* London: Jessica Kingsley Publishers

*Jackson, L. (2002). *Freaks, geeks and Asperger syndrome: a user guide to adolescence,* London: Jessica Kingsley Publishers

**Jones, G. (2001). Giving the diagnosis to the young person with Asperger syndrome or high functioning autism: issues and strategies, *Good Autism Practice,* 2, 2, p65- 71

*Murray, D. (2006). *Coming out Asperger,* London: Jessica Kingsley Publishers

**Newson, E. (2000). 'Writing to children and young people with Asperger syndrome,' *Good Autism Practice,* 1, 2, p17- 27

Paine, S. and Phillip, T. (2000). *Artists emerging: sustaining expression through drawing,* London: Lund Humphries

*Sainsbury, C. (2000). *Martian in the playground: understanding the schoolchild with Asperger's syndrome,* Bristol: Lucky Duck Publishing

*Available from the distributor of NAS Publications:
Central Books Ltd
99 Wallis Road
London E9 5LN
Tel: 0845 458 9911
Or order online @ www.autism.org.uk/pubs

**Available from NAS Information Centre
393 City Road,
London EC1V 1NG
Tel: 0845 070 4004
Photocopy request form from
http://www.autism.org.uk/infocentre
Or search for the articles on Autism Data
www.autism.org.uk/autismdata and select from there.

Talking together about an autism diagnosis

Useful resources

There are many books which aim to give more information about ASDs and what they might mean for individuals. Some books are aimed at the individuals themselves, some at brothers and sisters, some at parents/carers and some at professionals. It might be useful to have a look at several books to work out which words and style might be right for your child. It is often helpful to adapt what has been written by other people to make it suitable for your child.

For children and young people with an ASD

*Doherty, K., McNally, P. and Sherrard, E. (2000).
I have autism...what's that? Lisburn: Down Lisburn Trust
*Elder, J. (2006). *Different like me: my book of autism heroes.* London: Jessica Kingsley Publishers
*Gerland, G. (2000). *Finding out about Asperger syndrome, high-functioning autism and PDD.* London: Jessica Kingsley Publishers
*Jackson, L. (2002). *Freaks, Geeks and Asperger syndrome.* London: Jessica Kingsley Publishers
*NAS Autism Helpline (1999). *What is Asperger syndrome and how will it affect me?* London: The National Autistic Society

For other children

*Hannah, E. (2007). *My friend Sam: introducing a child with autism to a nursery school.* London: The National Autistic Society
*Peters, C. (2007). *That's not fair! Explaining autism to very young children.* Leicester: Leicester City Council
*Powell, J. (2006). *Thomas has autism,* London: Evans Brothers
Spilsbury, L. (2001). *What does it mean to have autism?* Oxford: Heinemann

For brothers and sisters

*Al-Ghani, H. (2007). *I really don't know why: a sibling song to autism.* London: The National Autistic Society
*Brock, C. (2007). *My family is different: a workbook for children with a brother or sister who has autism or Asperger syndrome.* London: The National Autistic Society
*Fairfoot, E. (2004). *My special brother Rory.* London: The National Autistic Society
*Gorrod, L. (1997). *My brother is different: a book for young children who have brothers and sisters.* London: The National Autistic Society
*Hunter, S.T. (2006). *My sister is different.* London: The National Autistic Society
*Koutsis, A. et al. (2006). *What about me? The autism survival guide for kids.* Australia: Wantirna High School
*Welton, J. (2003). *Can I tell you about Asperger syndrome? A guide for family and friends.* London: Jessica Kingsley Publishers

For adults

*Fleisher, M. (2003). *Making sense of the unfeasible: my life journey with Asperger syndrome.* London: Jessica Kingsley Publishers
Asperger United is a quarterly newsletter written mainly by people with Asperger syndrome for people with Asperger syndrome aged 16 or over. You can download the latest edition from the NAS website. To subscribe contact the NAS Publication Team on 0207 903 3595. Subscription is free.

Books aimed at parents and carers

*Murray, D. ed. (2006). *Coming out Asperger.* London: Jessica Kingsley Publishers

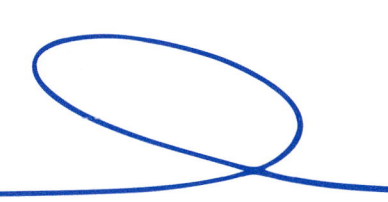

Work books

Faherty, C. (2000). *Asperger's…What does it mean to me?* Arlington: Future Horizons Inc.
*Kershaw, P. (2008). *Working together on autism.* London: The National Autistic Society.
*Vermeulen, P. (2000). *I am special: introducing children and young people to their autistic spectrum disorder.* Jessica Kingsley Publishers

Novels for children and young people which feature characters with an ASD

*Haddon, M. (2003). *The curious incident of the dog in the night-time.* London: David Fickling Books
*Hoopman, K. (2000) *Blue bottle mystery,* London: Jessica Kingsley Publishers
*Ogaz, N. (2004). *Wishing on the midnight star: my Asperger brother.* London: Jessica Kingsley Publishers
*Rees, C. (2000). *Truth or dare.* London: Macmillan
*Victor, P. (2006). *Baj and the word launcher: space age Asperger adventures in communication.* London: Jessica Kingsley Publishers
*Welton, J. (2004). *Adam's alternative sports day: an Asperger story.* London: Jessica Kingsley Publishers

DVDs

*Eye Television (2006). *A different life: Rosie's story.* Norwich: Eye Television
*Hoy, R. (2007). *Autism and me.* London: Jessica Kingsley Publishers
*Available from the distributor of NAS Publications:
Central Books Ltd
99 Wallis Road
London E9 5LN
Tel: 0845 458 9911
Fax: 0845 458 9912
Or order online @ www.autism.org.uk/pubs

Websites
General

> The National Autistic Society website has a huge range of information sheets, details of support groups, social groups, books, leaflets which could all be helpful:
www.autism.org.uk
> Carol Gray's website gives information about Social Stories™ with tips on how to write them and resources to buy:
www.thegraycenter.org

By young people for young people

> tqjunior.thinkquest.org/5852/autism.htm

For young people

> faculty.washington.edu/chudler/aut.html
> www.cdc.gov/ncbddd/kids/kautismpage.htm

Acknowledgements

With grateful thanks for contributions from the NAS *Help!* team, Jenny Rowbottom, formerly of the NAS press team for the lesson plans, and for the time and thoughts of Professor Anthony Bailey, Reece Scott Chair of Psychiatry, University of Oxford, and Sheila Coates, Chair, Children in Touch, former head of the Chinnor Resource Units in Oxfordshire, Carol Gray and Christine Deudney.

The author, Rachel Pike has worked for The National Autistic Society for a number of years as a Regional Officer in the south-west, north and midlands. She has many years practical experience of working with children, young people and adults with an ASD and their families. She is author of *Supporting students with Asperger syndrome in higher education*, also published by The National Autistic Society.

The illustrator, Jess Abbo, has worked for many years as a professional cartoonist and illustrator. He has illustrated a number of books for NAS Publications, including *Going to the doctor*, *Going on trips* and *Advocacy for adults with autism spectrum disorders: a guide*.